Fast Facts

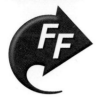

Fast Facts:
Osteoporosis

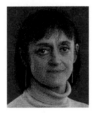

Juliet E Compston FRCP FRCPath FMedSci

Professor of Bone Medicine

University of Cambridge School of Clinical Medicine

and Consultant Physician

Addenbrooke's Hospital

Cambridge, UK

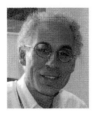

Clifford J Rosen MD

Senior Scientist

Maine Medical Center

Research Institute

Scarborough, Maine, USA

Declaration of Independence
This book is as balanced and as practical as we can make it.
Ideas for improvement are always welcome: feedback@fastfacts.com

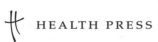

HEALTH PRESS

Fast Facts: Osteoporosis
First published 1997; second edition 1999; third edition 2002;
fourth edition 2004; fifth edition 2006
Sixth edition March 2009

Text © 2009 Juliet E Compston, Clifford J Rosen
© 2009 in this edition Health Press Limited
Health Press Limited, Elizabeth House, Queen Street, Abingdon,
Oxford OX14 3LN, UK
Tel: +44 (0)1235 523233
Fax: +44 (0)1235 523238

Book orders can be placed by telephone or via the website.
For regional distributors or to order via the website, please go to:
www.fastfacts.com
For telephone orders, please call +44 (0)1752 202301 (UK and Europe),
1 800 247 6553 (USA, toll free), +1 419 281 1802 (Americas) or
+61 (0)2 9351 6173 (Asia–Pacific).

Fast Facts is a trademark of Health Press Limited.

A CIP record for this title is available from the British Library.

ISBN 978-1-905832-51-4

The cover image is a composite BSE scanning electron microscopy image of a
parasagittal slice of L4 from 89-year-old female. Information from three 'overhead'
fast electron detectors was coded as red, green or blue components in order to create
the composite image. Color hue shows orientation and color intensity shows the slope
of the surface. Field, 4.24 mm wide and high. Sample, 2.8mm thick. Reproduced with
the permission of Professor Alan Boyde, Queen Mary, University of London, UK.

Compston JE (Juliet)
Fast Facts: Osteoporosis/
Juliet E Compston, Clifford J Rosen

Medical illustrations by Dee McLean, London, UK.
Typesetting and page layout by Zed, Oxford, UK.
Printed by Latimer Trend & Company Limited, Plymouth, UK.

Text printed with vegetable inks on biodegradable and
recyclable paper manufactured from sustainable forests.

Low
chlorine

Sustainable
forests

Glossary of abbreviations   4

Introduction   5

Epidemiology   7

Pathophysiology   12

Clinical manifestations   25

Diagnostic techniques   32

Risk assessment   45

Management: general considerations   52

Antiresorptive therapy   60

Strontium ranelate and parathyroid hormone peptides   78

Other forms of osteoporosis   85

Future trends   90

Useful addresses   96

Index   98

Glossary of abbreviations

Anabolic hormones: synthetic or natural hormones that stimulate bone remodeling, particularly by enhancing bone formation more than bone resorption

Antiresorptive drugs: hormonal or synthetic agents (including estrogens, raloxifene, bisphosphonates and calcitonin) that work by suppressing bone remodeling, particularly bone resorption

Bisphosphonates: drugs that bind to bone mineral with antiresorptive properties

BMD: bone mineral density

BMU: bone multicellular (or remodeling) unit

Calcitonin: a naturally occurring polypeptide that inhibits bone resorption

DXA: dual-energy X-ray absorptiometry

HRT: hormone replacement therapy

Osteoblast: a cell responsible for the formation of bone

Osteoclast: a large multinuclear cell that resorbs bone

Osteogenesis imperfecta: an inherited disorder of collagen characterized by bones that fracture easily

Osteomalacia: softening of bones caused by a loss of mineral, usually due to a deficiency in vitamin D

PTH: parathyroid hormone

QUS: quantitative ultrasound

SERM: selective estrogen-receptor modulator

T-score: standard deviation score related to mean reference value for peak bone mass

Z-score: standard deviation score related to mean reference value for age-matched bone mineral density

Introduction

The diagnosis and treatment of osteoporosis has been revolutionized in the past decade. The technology for imaging trabecular and cortical bone has improved dramatically through the use of magnetic resonance imaging and quantitative computed tomography (CT). Utilization of bone mineral density (BMD) measurements to assess the risk of fracture has grown exponentially. However, the identification of high-risk individuals for treatment has now been significantly improved by the FRAX™ risk-assessment tool. This online algorithm, supported by the World Health Organization, enables clinicians to estimate the 10-year probability of major osteoporotic fracture using clinical risk factors with or without BMD measurements. Bone quality has taken on a new meaning in light of studies using dual-energy X-ray absorptiometry and CT together. Markers of bone turnover, another indicator of risk, have become more precise and are now easier to use and interpret.

On the treatment side, the results of large randomized trials have broadened our perspective on therapies for preventing and treating this condition. New bisphosphonates with reduced dosing frequency have been approved; the most recent of these, zoledronate, requires only once yearly administration. Parathyroid hormone (PTH) peptides have emerged as exciting new options for building bone mass and preventing devastating fractures in severely osteoporotic individuals. Newer means of administering PTH or altering the frequency of administration may lead to wider utilization of a relatively safe but expensive intervention. Similarly, strontium ranelate has been found to be effective in reducing fractures. New selective estrogen-receptor molecules are being developed and are likely to be approved in the future. Hormone replacement has beneficial effects on the skeleton, but these are outweighed in older postmenopausal women by several adverse outcomes, including a greater risk of stroke and breast cancer. Calcium and vitamin D supplementation is probably useful as an adjunct in patients with established osteoporosis, but its role as global preventive therapy for all postmenopausal women has been questioned by several recent randomized controlled trials.

Thus, this sixth edition of *Fast Facts: Osteoporosis* highlights recent developments in the therapeutic and diagnostic arena, while maintaining the background sections that clarify the pathophysiology of osteoporosis and the homeostatic determinants of peak bone acquisition and maintenance.

As we have maintained from the beginning, family physicians and healthcare professionals play a key role in diagnosing, preventing and treating this disease. In spite of substantial advances in the identification of high-risk individuals and the emergence of new treatments, many patients with fractures still do not receive appropriate management. Successful bridging of this care gap requires keen awareness of risk factors amongst healthcare professionals and the lay public alike, better communication between secondary and primary care, and more widespread use of appropriate therapeutic interventions. Poor adherence to osteoporosis therapy provides a major challenge that may be addressed by better patient education and follow-up in primary care. We believe this book will help all clinicians achieve this goal.

Osteoporosis is a major cause of illness and death in the elderly. The condition is characterized by low bone mass (Figure 1.1), which increases the risk of fracture, particularly of the spine, hip and wrist.

Of people surviving to 80 years of age, 1 in 3 women and 1 in 5 men will suffer a hip fracture. These so-called 'fragility' fractures result in annual costs estimated at £2.1 billion in the UK, €25 billion in Europe and US$19 billion in the USA. In women, the hospital costs for osteoporotic fractures exceed those for stroke and myocardial infarction (Figure 1.2).

Fractures

The total number of fractures attributable to osteoporosis each year is estimated at 250 000 in the UK and 1.5 million in the USA. Worldwide, it is estimated that 200 million women suffer from osteoporosis. By the age of 50, the lifetime risk of a fracture due to osteoporosis in a white woman is nearly 40%, similar to the lifetime risk for coronary heart

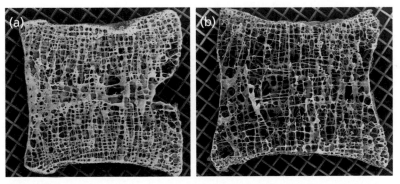

Figure 1.1 Scanning electron micrograph images of 4 mm-thick slices of lumbar vertebrae (vertebral bodies) from (a) a young person and (b) an elderly person, showing the reduction in bone mass and loss of bone structure associated with aging. The samples are resting on a 2.33 periodicity wire mesh grid. Reproduced with the permission of Professor Alan Boyde, Queen Mary, University of London, UK.

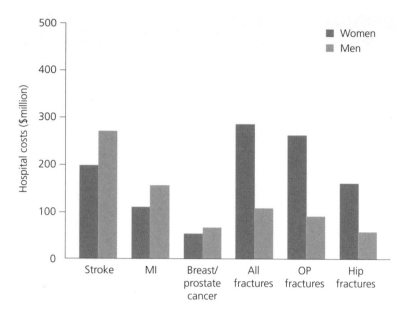

Figure 1.2 Hospital costs attributable to different diseases in Sweden. In women, the costs for treating osteoporotic (OP) fractures are greater than those for treating stroke, myocardial infarction (MI) or breast cancer. The number of bed days occupied by women with OP fractures also exceeds the number attributable to stroke and heart disease (data not shown). Adapted from Johnell et al. 2005.

disease; in men, the corresponding figure is 13% (see Osteoporosis in men, page 87) (Figure 1.3).

In the UK, there are an estimated 60 000 hip fractures, 50 000 fractures of the radius and 40 000 clinically diagnosed vertebral fractures each year; in the USA, the corresponding figures are 300 000, 500 000 and 200 000.

In Europe, approximately 179 000 men and 611 000 women suffer a hip fracture each year, while 11.5% and 35% of women aged 50–54 years and 75–79 years, respectively, have at least one vertebral fracture. Other fragility fractures, particularly those of the pelvis and humerus, are also a significant cause of morbidity in the elderly.

The incidence of osteoporotic fractures increases markedly with age (Figure 1.4). In women, this increase is seen after the age of 45 years and

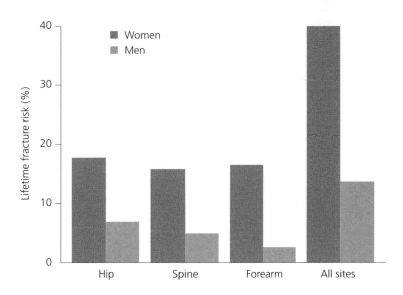

Figure 1.3 Estimated lifetime risk of fragility fracture for 50-year-old white women and men. Adapted from data in Melton LJ 3rd et al. *J Bone Miner Res* 1992;7:1005–10.

is mainly due to forearm fractures up to the age of 65 years, after which the incidence of hip fractures rises exponentially. In men, the incidence of fragility fractures increases after the age of 75 years.

The hip is the most common fracture site in both sexes after the age of 85 years. The incidence of vertebral fractures is less well documented, but for clinically diagnosed fractures there is an exponential increase with age in men and a more linear age-related increase in women.

There are marked geographic variations in the incidence of osteoporotic fractures, partly because of racial differences in skeletal size; osteoporosis is most common in Asian and white populations, and rare in African-American black populations. In many parts of the world, there is evidence that osteoporotic fractures have become more common in recent decades, even after allowing for the aging population. Although this age-specific increase may now be stabilizing in some countries, the increase in life expectancy alone is likely to at least double the number of hip fractures over the next 50 years.

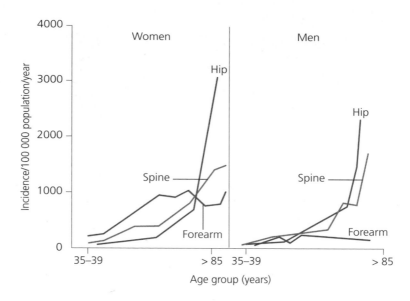

Figure 1.4 Incidence of hip, forearm and clinically diagnosed spinal fractures in women and men at different ages. Reprinted from Cooper C, Melton LJ. *Trends Endocrin Metab* 1992;3:224–9, with permission from Elsevier. Copyright © 1992.

Key points – epidemiology

- Osteoporosis increases the risk of fragility fractures, particularly in the hip, wrist and spine.
- The incidence of osteoporosis rises rapidly with age.
- Of people surviving to 80 years of age, 1 in 3 women and 1 in 5 men will suffer a hip fracture.
- The number of osteoporotic fractures is expected to at least double over the next few decades as a result of demographic changes.
- Fragility fractures impose a huge economic burden on healthcare services.

Key references

Cole ZA, Dennison EM, Cooper C. Osteoporosis epidemiology update. *Curr Rheumatol Rep* 2008;10:92–6.

Cummings SR, Melton LJ 3rd. Epidemiology and outcomes of osteoporotic fractures. *Lancet* 2002;359:1761–7.

Johnell O, Kanis JA, Jonsson B et al. The burden of hospitalised fractures in Sweden. *Osteoporos Int* 2005; 16:222–8.

Khosla S, Amin S, Orwoll E. Osteoporosis in men. *Endocr Rev* 2008;29:441–64

Melton LJ 3rd, Lane AW, Cooper C et al. Prevalence and incidence of vertebral deformities. *Osteoporos Int* 1993;3:113–19.

van Staa TP, Dennison EM, Leufkens HG, Cooper C. Epidemiology of fractures in England and Wales. *Bone* 2001;29:517–22.

Low bone mineral density (BMD, also referred to as bone mass) is one of the most important predisposing factors for osteoporotic fractures.

Adult BMD is determined both by the acquisition of peak bone mass during adolescence and the degree of subsequent bone loss (Figure 2.1). These two processes are regulated at the level of the bone remodeling units, which, in turn, are governed by genetic and environmental factors.

An osteoporotic fracture occurs as a result of trauma – major or minor – to a bone that has reduced bone quantity and quality. Although there is a strong inverse relationship between BMD and fracture risk, other mechanical factors are important for defining bone strength and hence absolute fracture risk. Such determinants are difficult to assess clinically, and are often referred to as qualitative risk factors. These include rate of bone turnover, trabecular connectivity, cortical and trabecular thickness, bone shape and the structural model index (a measure of the platelike consistency of bone). Recent efforts have focused on in vivo measurements for these determinants using quantitative computed tomography and magnetic resonance imaging (MRI).

Notwithstanding the issues surrounding bone quality, it is clear that the lower the BMD, the less force is necessary to produce a fracture. Falls that result in soft-tissue and skeletal injury are therefore critical in the pathogenesis of osteoporotic fractures (see Figure 2.1), and therapeutic intervention must aim both to prevent bone loss and to reduce the likelihood of falls.

It now seems certain that fractures in virtually every skeletal site in postmenopausal women can be considered osteoporotic in nature, the only exception being facial fractures and compound injuries due to motor vehicle accidents.

Bone remodeling

A knowledge of the process of bone remodeling is important in order to understand how bone mass can be altered by heritable and environmental influences. Skeletal remodeling, which predominates

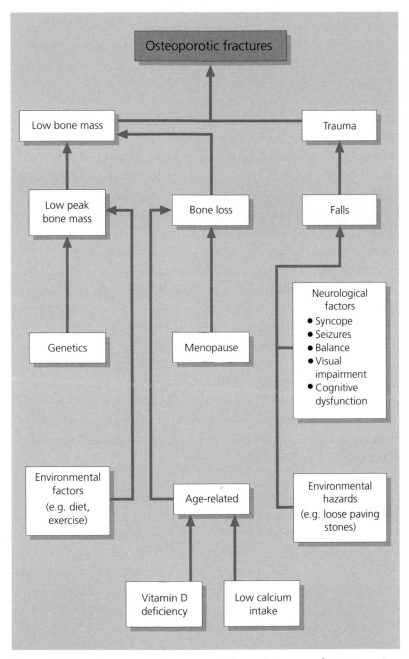

Figure 2.1 Low bone mass plus trauma is the major cause of osteoporotic fractures.

once longitudinal growth ceases, occurs in bone 'multicellular' units (BMUs). It begins with bone dissolution or resorption and ends with new bone formation.

Bone resorption is carried out by cells called osteoclasts, which originate from the monocyte–macrophage lineage. New bone is formed by osteoblasts, cells of the fibroblast–stromal lineage that produce several bone matrix proteins and synthesize a lattice for subsequent mineralization. Osteocytes are old osteoblasts that have become entombed within the bone matrix. Although not actively dividing, these cells are connected to lining cells on the endosteal surface of bone through tiny canaliculi. It is thought that osteocytes can sense changes in gravitational forces and loading, and in this way initiate, via the canaliculi, signals that activate osteoblasts and osteoclasts.

In adulthood, each remodeling cycle is balanced – resorption equals formation – and lasts between 90 and 130 days (Figure 2.2). Maintenance of bone mass during remodeling ensures a ready source of calcium for the body and a persistent reservoir of stored calcium. However, remodeling cycles can become imbalanced, and over several cycles this can result in significant bone loss. These imbalances are almost always a result of greater bone resorption relative to bone formation and can often be traced to changes in systemic hormones, dietary intake or mechanical loading. An unsteady state in the BMUs leads to bone loss and diminution in mechanical strength, resulting in diminished bone quality and quantity.

Peak bone mass

Most bone mass is acquired during childhood and adolescence when modeling of the skeleton is at its peak and remodeling favors the formation of bone, thereby permitting a significant and critical increase in bone mass. In general, peak bone mass is attained by 20 years of age (Figure 2.3), with peak trabecular bone mass being attained at around 12–16 years of age (depending on gender) and peak cortical bone mass being attained at around 20–24 years of age.

Longitudinal studies of bone acquisition in adolescents have shown that several factors regulate peak bone density; the most important of these are genetic determinants.

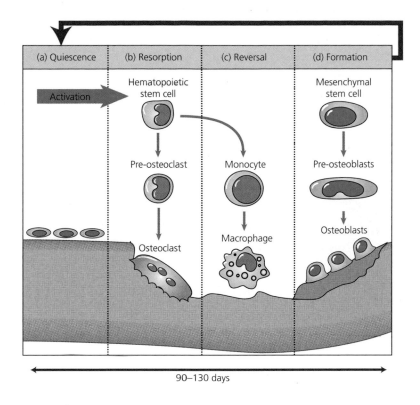

90–130 days

Figure 2.2 Bone remodeling is a balanced, orderly process. (a) Quiescence – in this resting state, the bone surface is covered with flattened lining cells. (b) Resorption – osteoclasts remove bone mineral and matrix, creating an erosion cavity. (c) Reversal – mononuclear cells prepare the bone surface for new osteoblasts to begin building bone. (d) Formation – osteoblasts synthesize an organic matrix to replace resorbed bone and fill the cavity with new bone.

Despite intense efforts over the past decade, the heritable determinants of bone mass, although clearly important, have not been identified. Nevertheless, recent work in humans and in mice has identified two new signaling pathways that are genetically regulated:
- the *Wnt/LRP5/β-catenin* canonical (lipoprotein receptor-related protein 5) signaling network
- the lipoxygenase pathway.

15

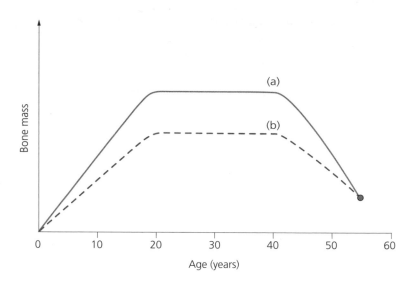

Figure 2.3 Peak bone mass is attained by the age of 20 years. Low bone mass at 50–60 years of age can be due to either (a) accelerated bone loss or (b) low peak bone mass.

In the former pathway, activating mutations of the membrane-bound *LRP5* cause high bone mass; conversely, inactivating mutations lead to osteoporosis pseudoganglioma syndrome, a condition associated with low bone mass and blindness in children. Families with the 'high bone mass' gene have been identified and are characterized by extremely high BMD measurements (T-scores of +2.0 to +5.0) in most skeletal sites. Members of these families are healthy, with structurally sound bone and normal markers of bone turnover. It is hypothesized that high bone mass results from enhanced mechanical sensing.

In the lipoxygenase pathway, two critical enzyme-regulating genes determine when and how bone-marrow stromal cells enter the fat or bone lineage: 12, 15 *lipoxygenase* (12-LO or *Alox 12, 15*), which produces prostaglandins and other endogenous ligands that bind to the peroxisome proliferator-activated receptor gamma (PPARγ), a nuclear receptor that induces adipocyte differentiation at the expense of osteoblast formation; and 5-LO or *Alox 5*, which generates leukotrienes that can also activate PPARγ and influence stromal cell differentiation.

Polymorphisms in these two genes in mice and humans have been associated with marked differences in peak bone mass. More studies are under way to fully appreciate these and other signaling networks necessary for optimal bone acquisition.

It now seems likely that there are important polymorphisms in many genes that regulate bone acquisition, including the above-mentioned pathway genes and others such as the vitamin-D receptor, estrogen receptor, parathyroid hormone receptor, insulin-like growth factor-I and collagen type 1, alpha 1. Interestingly, many genes that work within a given network are also located in blocks within the human genome, suggesting that heritable influences include evolutionary changes in several genes, which result in altered susceptibility to diseases such as osteoporosis.

Environmental determinants interact with genetic influences to modify acquisition of peak bone mass. The most important non-heritable factors are:

- sex steroid and growth hormone production
- calcium intake
- physical activity.

All three factors have been shown in randomized or observational trials to influence the velocity and zenith of peak bone acquisition.

With respect to calcium intake, supplemental calcium given to young girls entering puberty enhances their rate of bone acquisition compared with placebo, although in late adolescence, those with lower calcium intakes eventually reach the same BMD as those receiving supplements.

Weight-bearing exercise can enhance bone mass by 1–2% per year during adolescence. Absence or mistiming of the growth spurt, and delays in menarche, result in a lower final adult bone mass.

Factors influencing bone mass

In adults, bone mass at any given time is the sum of two factors: peak bone mass and the rate of current and past bone loss. For example, the measured bone mass of a 52-year-old woman would be the result of:

- bone acquisition during childhood and adolescence
- ongoing or previous bone loss (possibly as a result of the menopause).

TABLE 2.1

Risk factors for osteoporosis

- Hypogonadism (including premature menopause)
- Glucocorticoid therapy
- Previous fracture, particularly after menopause
- Low bodyweight
- Current cigarette smoking
- Excess alcohol consumption
- Low dietary calcium intake
- Vitamin D deficiency
- Late puberty
- Physical inactivity
- High caffeine intake
- Maternal history of hip fracture
- Other secondary causes of osteoporosis (see Table 4.4)

Although persistent bone loss is a feature in most patients with osteoporosis, impaired acquisition of peak bone mass is responsible for 60–70% of the variance in bone mass at any age. Hormonal and environmental factors remain the strongest determinants of bone loss after the fourth decade in both men and women, whereas heritable influences, sex hormone status and dietary calcium are the principal regulators of peak bone mass.

Several risk factors are associated with osteoporosis (Table 2.1), each of which may influence peak bone mass and the rate of bone loss, resulting in reduced bone mass. However, a bone mass measurement will predict the risk of fracture more accurately than calculation of risk factor scores other than a previous fracture (see below).

Bone loss

Hormonal influences. During the menopause, estrogen deprivation enhances the rate of bone dissolution, and most women experience bone loss of, on average, about 1% per year; however, in a small proportion of women, loss of spine BMD can be as great as 5% per year.

It is not possible to identify women with bone loss prospectively. Although bone formation is accelerated in an attempt to match higher rates of resorption during menopause, the time required for bone formation does not permit this process to completely match resorption. The result is a net loss of bone (Figure 2.4). For example, a 45-year-old woman with early menopause is at increased risk of osteoporotic fractures because of the accelerated bone loss that occurs after estrogen deprivation. In contrast, the increased risk in a 50-year-old woman with a strong family history of osteoporosis is mainly caused by impaired acquisition of peak bone mass (see Figure 2.3).

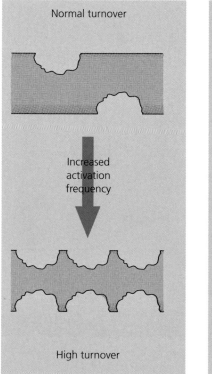
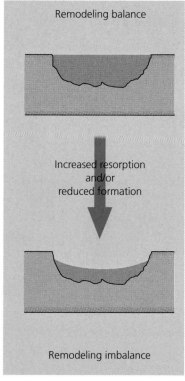

Figure 2.4 Osteoporosis is the result of an increase in the number of remodeling cycles, and/or an imbalance within each bone remodeling unit, resulting in a net loss of bone.

Young amenorrheic athletes are at even higher risk of osteoporosis because of both impaired acquisition of peak bone mass and accelerated bone loss.

Age-associated bone loss. In the elderly, age-associated bone loss results from chronic 'uncoupling', or an imbalance, of resorption and formation. Resorption is normal or increased, but bone formation is suppressed, unchanged or only slightly increased. Chronic imbalance leads to persistent bone loss and an increased risk of future fracture (Figure 2.5). Other factors besides estrogen (or androgen) deprivation can produce bone loss in the elderly.

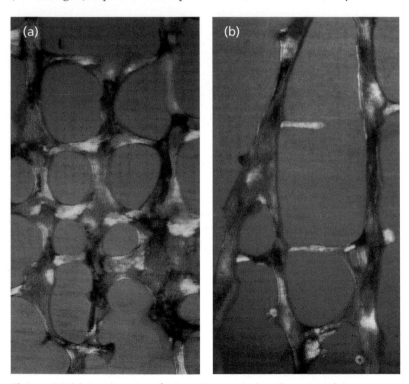

Figure 2.5 (a) An almost perfect continuous trabecular network in a 50-year-old man compared with (b) thinned horizontal trabeculae and wider separation of the vertical structure in a 76-year-old man. Reprinted from Mosekilde L. *Bone* 1998;9:247–50. Copyright © 1988, with permission from Elsevier.

Calcium or vitamin D deficiency and secondary hyperparathyroidism can account for bone resorption rates that equal or exceed menopausal levels. In addition, recent evidence suggests that marrow adiposity increases with age, and is an independent risk factor for fracture. MRI has demonstrated the presence of significant fat in the marrow of older individuals; although the reasons for this are not known, an inverse relationship between marrow fat and BMD has been demonstrated. There is some evidence that a default mechanism is activated when pre-osteoblasts are unable to enter the bone lineage, but it remains to be determined whether this is related to the PPARγ/lipoxygenase or Wnt signaling pathways. On the other hand, there is also indirect evidence that marrow fat may be an important energy depot for residual osteoblasts that are hyperfunctioning due to greatly increased apoptosis of mature osteoblasts.

Although older people tend to consume less calcium, there are other factors that also contribute to a state of relative calcium deficiency. In particular, aging is associated with reduced synthesis of 1,25-dihydroxyvitamin D, the active metabolite of vitamin D, and reduced production of a major precursor of vitamin D in the skin. The reduction in these vitamin D compounds contributes to lower calcium absorption, which leads to increased secretion of parathyroid hormone and enhanced bone resorption.

Glucocorticoids. One of the most common causes of osteoporosis in both men and women is glucocorticoid-induced bone loss. Glucocorticoids have a profound effect on the skeleton by simultaneously suppressing bone formation and enhancing bone resorption, in a dose-dependent manner. Furthermore, secondary hyperparathyroidism often results from impaired calcium absorption. These events lead to uncoupling in the remodeling sequence (Figure 2.6) and result in rapid bone loss, particularly during the first 6–12 months of glucocorticoid therapy.

Randomized, placebo-controlled trials have firmly established the efficacy of bisphosphonates in the prevention and treatment of glucocorticoid-induced osteoporosis (see pages 85–7).

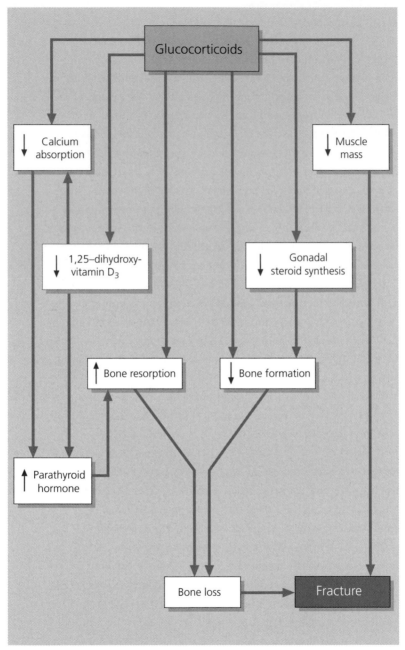

Figure 2.6 Glucocorticoid therapy causes bone loss by suppressing bone formation and increasing bone resorption.

Immunosuppressant therapy. Use of other immunosuppressants, such as ciclosporin, can further exacerbate steroid-induced bone loss. In addition to the loss of bone mass that results from chronic glucocorticoid use, patients taking long-term steroids have an increased risk of vertebral and non-vertebral fractures. These events are also dose- and time-dependent but are more common in postmenopausal women.

Other factors. Excess levels of thyroid hormone and chronic anticonvulsant therapy also increase bone loss. A very high protein intake may be deleterious to bone since it increases urinary calcium excretion, whereas alkali foods such as fruit and vegetables have been shown to have beneficial effects. However, the magnitude of these effects remains unclear. Hematologic factors may also be associated with secondary causes of osteoporosis. Malignancies such as myeloma, lymphoma and leukemia, in which local cytokines are released directly into the bone marrow, can lead to increased bone resorption, osteopenia diagnosed by densitometry, lytic lesions apparent on radiographic film and osteoporotic fractures. Metastatic neoplasms to bone can also cause regional bone loss and fractures.

Key points – pathophysiology

- Bone density measurements strongly predict fracture risk, but bone quality is also a determinant of bone strength; measuring bone quality in vivo requires sophisticated tools, such as magnetic resonance imaging and quantitative computed tomography.
- Peak bone mass is a critical determinant of adult bone density; 60% of peak bone mass is determined by genetic factors that have not yet been identified.
- Menopause is associated with bone loss; some menopausal women lose bone rapidly (> 5% per year), while others lose bone at a rate of approximately 1% per year.
- Age-related bone loss is accelerated by impaired calcium intake and low levels of vitamin D.

Key references

Bouxsein ML. Bone quality: where do we go from here? *Osteoporos Int* 2003;14(suppl 5):118–27.

Cummings SR, Nevitt MC, Browner WS et al. Risk factors for hip fracture in white women. Study of Osteoporotic Fractures Research Group. *N Engl J Med* 1995; 332:767–73.

Greenspan SL, Myers ER, Kiel DP et al. Fall direction, bone mineral density, and function: risk factors for hip fracture in frail nursing home elderly. *Am J Med* 1998;104:539–45.

Guyatt GH, Cranney A, Griffith L et al. Summary of meta-analyses of therapies for postmenopausal osteoporosis and the relationship between bone density and fractures. *Endocrinol Metab Clin North Am* 2002;31:659–79.

Khosla S, Melton LJ 3rd, Atkinson EJ, O'Fallon WM. Relationship of serum sex steroid levels to longitudinal changes in bone density in young versus elderly men. *J Clin Endocrinol Metab* 2001; 86:3555–61.

Klein RF, Allard J, Avnur Z et al. Regulation of bone mass in mice by the lipoxygenase gene Alox15. *Science* 2004;303:229–32.

Little RD, Carulli JP, Del Mastro RG et al. A mutation in the LDL receptor-related protein 5 gene results in the autosomal dominant high-bone-mass trait. *Am J Hum Genet* 2002;70:11–19.

Manolagas SC. Birth and death of bone cells: basic regulatory mechanisms and implications for the pathogenesis and treatment of osteoporosis. *Endocr Rev* 2000;21:115–37.

Recker RR, Heaney RP. Peak bone mineral density in young women. *JAMA* 1993;270:2926–7.

Storm D, Eslin R, Porter ES et al. Calcium supplementation prevents seasonal bone loss and changes in biochemical markers of bone turnover in elderly New England women: a randomized placebo-controlled trial. *J Clin Endocrinol Metab* 1998;83:3817–25.

Osteoporosis is a silent disease until a fracture is sustained. Before this, bone loss or failure to attain peak bone mass is not associated with any signs or symptoms. Measuring bone mineral density (BMD) is the most accurate way to determine whether bone mass has been compromised. Apart from this, however, the main clinical presentations of osteoporosis are:

- fragility/low trauma fracture
- pain
- height loss
- incidental osteopenia reported during a radiological examination.

In patients with these presentations, the disease process has already progressed significantly. For example, a low bone mass detected by conventional radiographs (taken for other reasons) usually equates to a bone mass 3–4 standard deviations below the young normal mean.

Initial presentation

Fractures of the wrist or spine are the principal presenting signs of osteoporosis in younger postmenopausal women, while hip fractures are more common in the elderly. In women aged 45–65 years, a Colles' fracture of the wrist, produced by impaction of the distal head of the radius, is commonly the first visible manifestation of osteoporosis. Often, however, the patient and physician will attribute the injury to a fall, without considering the possibility of osteoporosis. Spinal fractures, on the other hand, may present with severe mid-thoracic or lower back pain without a history of trauma. In up to two-thirds of patients in whom compression fractures are diagnosed radiographically, the patient cannot recall a traumatic event. In the remaining one-third, however, acute back pain due to compression fractures can often be related to mild or moderate trauma.

Generally, the lower the bone mass, the lower the trauma necessary to incur a fracture. Thus, in very severe osteoporosis, a rib or thoracic spine fracture can be sustained after coughing, or rolling over in bed.

Once again, a detailed patient history, including a description of daily routines, will often provide clues to the type of injury sustained. This information is critical for patient management, as the patient or carer can then be given advice about changing the level of physical activity in order to avoid future fractures.

Spinal fractures

Acute onset of back pain in a woman with a history of spinal fracture often indicates a new fracture. The relative risk of a new vertebral fracture is:

- more than doubled in a patient with a previous vertebral fracture
- more than quadrupled in a patient with a previous vertebral fracture combined with low bone mass.

These new fractures often occur rapidly after the initial one, so that a woman who has just sustained a vertebral fracture has a one-in-five chance of suffering another within the next 12 months.

Several types of spinal fracture can occur (Figure 3.1). Diagnosis of a new vertebral fracture is usually made on lateral spine radiographs (see Figure 4.5, page 40), and may be facilitated by

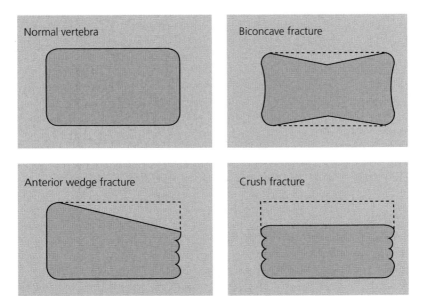

Figure 3.1 Types of vertebral fracture.

comparing current radiographs with previous ones, if available. Recently, attention has been drawn to the poor detection rate of vertebral fractures on spine radiographs. Even when detected, they are often not reported accurately. Occasionally, a technetium (99Tc) bone scan will illuminate areas in the spine in which a recent compression fracture has occurred. These areas may be undetectable on normal radiographic film. Dual-energy X-ray absorptiometry systems can also be used to diagnose vertebral fractures (see Chapter 4, Diagnostic techniques).

In addition to causing pain in some patients, vertebral fractures can result in:

- spinal deformity (kyphosis; Figure 3.2)
- height loss
- reduced physical mobility
- loss of self-esteem.

In severe cases there may also be respiratory symptoms, and abdominal pain due to contact between the lower ribs and the upper surface of the pelvis. Like hip fractures (see below), vertebral fractures are also associated with increased mortality, mainly as a result of comorbid conditions.

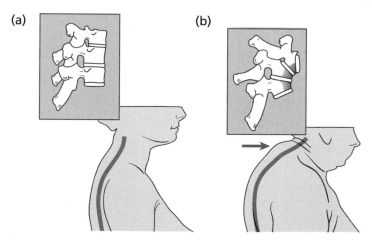

Figure 3.2 (a) Normal vertebrae. (b) Spinal deformity (kyphosis) caused by osteoporotic compression fractures of the thoracic spine. Note the so-called 'dowager's hump' (arrowed).

Hip fractures

Hip fractures are often the presenting manifestation of osteoporosis in elderly people. Osteopenia of the femur may be revealed by plain radiographs, and in some instances the orthopedic surgeon may comment on the fragility of bone at the time of surgery. Most patients with hip fractures are well over 70 years of age, and often have a low BMD, reduced body mass index, poor balance and slow reactions; many are also receiving multiple medications.

Occasionally, a traumatic hip fracture is the first clinical sign of neoplastic disease that has metastasized to the bone, and this possibility should be excluded during diagnosis (see Chapter 4, Diagnostic techniques).

Hip fractures are generally of three types (Figure 3.3):

- intertrochanteric
- femoral neck
- subcapital.

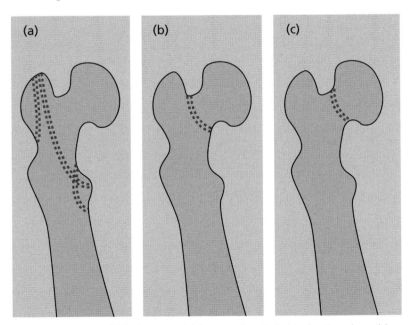

Figure 3.3 Types of hip fracture: (a) intertrochanteric hip fracture (possible sites); (b) basilar femoral neck fracture (undisplaced); (c) subcapital fracture (undisplaced).

In more than 90% of patients, hip fracture is caused by a fall. The type of fracture sustained depends on several factors, including the angle of fall, the type of fall (e.g. trip, slip or twist), the amount of protection afforded by subcutaneous fat and the patient's neuromuscular protective responses to the injury.

Wrist fractures

Fractures of the distal radius (Colles' fractures) are 10 times more common in women than men, and occur most often in women aged between 45 and 65 years, typically after a fall forwards onto the outstretched hand. Patients usually require one reduction (occasionally two), with 4–6 weeks in plaster to enable bone reunion. Most cases are treated as outpatients, although some older patients may require hospitalization. Some patients experience prolonged discomfort, often with a degree of disability, and deformity may develop as a result of malunion.

Other fractures

Other fractures associated with osteoporosis include proximal humeral, pelvic, distal tibia or tibia/fibula, and rib or tibia plateau fractures. At each of these bone sites there is a predominance of trabecular as opposed to cortical bone. This is significant, because during states of increased bone turnover such sites are particularly susceptible to bone loss and therefore more prone to injury. Fractures of mainly cortical sites (e.g. the metatarsals or proximal radius) are less common.

Short-term management

The orthopedic management of most osteoporotic fractures does not differ from that of other types of fracture in healthy individuals. Surgical stabilization is the mainstay of therapy, with special attention being paid during the postoperative period to determine and treat the underlying metabolic disorder.

Vertebral compression fractures are usually treated medically, with pain relief given as additional support. With this type of fracture, the pain is often intense for several weeks, and occasionally patients have to be hospitalized in order to treat complications, such as ileus or pneumonia. In acute cases with severe pain, vertebroplasty or kyphoplasty may be considered. These techniques involve the injection of bone cement into the fractured vertebra.

Narcotics and non-steroidal anti-inflammatory drugs are useful adjunctive therapy, along with gradual ambulation and physical therapy.

Back braces are ineffective in most patients, and tend to reduce the important effect of gravity on the skeleton (weight-bearing physical activity in which the body has to work against gravity helps to strengthen bones).

Physiotherapy, using measures such as hydrotherapy and transcutaneous electrical nerve stimulation (TENS), is often helpful in reducing pain.

Treatment with salmon calcitonin, administered either intranasally or by subcutaneous injection, can reduce bone pain and can therefore be used to lower the dose of narcotics needed to make the patient comfortable.

Epidural injection of glucocorticoids can also give dramatic pain relief in some patients and should be considered for patients hospitalized with intractable pain.

Long-term consequences

The long-term consequences of any osteoporotic fracture can be devastating. Approximately 20% of patients with hip fracture die within 6 months, and those who survive face a long and complicated rehabilitation. Vertebral fractures are also associated with increased mortality. For the elderly, the chance of regaining their original lifestyle is significantly reduced, and for patients with fractures of the spine, chronic pain and further fractures often follow.

Quality of life and physical activities can be significantly affected. Moreover, as patients with one spinal fracture are at greatly increased risk of further fractures, it is important to adopt an aggressive strategy for preventative treatment: bone-protective therapy should be considered even during the acute episode of pain. In general, the management of clinically evident osteoporosis should include a thorough evaluation of lifestyle, activity, diet and treatable risk factors, as well as measurement of BMD. Attention to risk factors for falling is especially important in frail elderly individuals. Adopting a comprehensive approach such as this will help to prevent future fractures and minimize future morbidity.

Key points – clinical manifestations

- Colles' (wrist) fractures occur mainly in young postmenopausal women following a fall onto the outstretched hand.
- Many vertebral fractures are asymptomatic and cannot be linked to preceding trauma.
- Only approximately one-third of vertebral fractures come to medical attention.
- Sequelae of spinal fractures include pain, spinal deformity, height loss, restriction of activity and loss of self-esteem.
- Hip fractures mainly occur in the frail elderly and are associated with a mortality of up to 20% at 6 months.
- Only one-third of patients with hip fractures regain their former level of independence.

Key references

Center JR, Nguyen TV, Schneider D et al. Mortality after all major types of osteoporotic fracture in men and women: an observational study. *Lancet* 1999;353:878–82.

Francis RM, Baillie SP, Chuck AJ et al. Acute and long-term management of patients with vertebral fractures. *QJM* 2004;97:63–74.

Gehlbach SH, Bigelow C, Heimisdottir M et al. Recognition of vertebral fracture in a clinical setting. *Osteoporos Int* 2000;11: 577–82.

Lindsay R, Silverman SL, Cooper C et al. Risk of new vertebral fracture in the year following a fracture. *JAMA* 2001;285:320–3.

Pluijm SM, Tromp AM, Smit JH et al. Consequences of vertebral deformities in older men and women. *J Bone Miner Res* 2000;15:1564–72.

Taylor RS, Fritzell P, Taylor RJ. Balloon kyphoplasty in the management of vertebral compression fractures: an updated systematic review and meta-analysis. *Eur Spine J* 2007;16:1085–100.

In recent years, there have been major advances in the diagnosis of osteoporosis. In particular, the measurement of bone mass at potential fracture sites by bone densitometry enables bone loss to be detected before fracture has occurred. This chapter examines the techniques and equipment used to evaluate bone mineral density (BMD), while the association between BMD and fracture risk is discussed in Chapter 5.

History and examination

A careful history and examination should be performed in all patients suspected of having osteoporosis. It is important to assess the clinical and historical risk factors (see Table 2.1, page 18), and to look for evidence of previous fragility fractures. Although the physical examination is often normal, the presence of dorsal kyphosis and restricted, painful spinal movements may indicate spinal osteoporosis.

Some forms of osteogenesis imperfecta, a rare cause of osteoporosis, are associated with blue sclerae. The patient should also be examined for clinical evidence of secondary causes of osteoporosis, such as malignancy or hyperthyroidism.

Bone densitometry

A number of techniques are now available to measure bone mass at various skeletal sites (Table 4.1). These techniques assist the assessment of fracture risk and have an established role in clinical practice (see Chapter 5, Risk assessment). The values obtained from these measurements represent the BMD.

BMD values are expressed as absolute values in g/cm^2 (i.e. as an areal density corrected for height or width of the bone but not depth) or as standard deviations (SDs) from the young adult (T-scores) or age-matched (Z-scores) reference range. Because different absorptiometers may give different absolute values for a given BMD measurement, the most widely employed diagnostic criteria for osteopenia and osteoporosis are based on SDs derived from reference data obtained in

TABLE 4.1

Methods for measurement of bone mineral density

Method	Sites measured
Dual-energy X-ray absorptiometry	Axial and appendicular skeleton, spine, femur, radius
Single-energy X-ray absorptiometry	Forearm, calcaneus
Quantitative computed tomography	Spine, femur, radius
Quantitative ultrasound	Calcaneus, patella

TABLE 4.2

Definitions of osteoporosis and osteopenia based on T-score and fracture history (defined by World Health Organization 1994)

T-score	Previous fragility	Classification fracture
Above −1	−	Normal
−1 to −2.5	−	Osteopenia
Below −2.5	−	Osteoporosis, with high risk of fracture
Below −2.5	≥1	Established osteoporosis

T-score, the number of standard deviations from the young normal adult mean bone mineral density; 'young normal' is defined as a population of healthy, white women aged 20–40 years.

premenopausal women (T-scores; Table 4.2, Figure 4.1). These criteria were developed for spine and/or hip BMD in postmenopausal women. However, they are likely also to apply to men, though there is still some uncertainty about whether the T-scores used should be derived from female or male reference data.

Osteopenia or osteoporosis, as defined in Table 4.2, may be found at one site of measurement in the presence of a normal BMD elsewhere in the skeleton. A diagnosis of osteoporosis (T-score ≤ 2.5) indicates a high risk of fracture; however, the greatest number of fractures occurs in individuals with osteopenia.

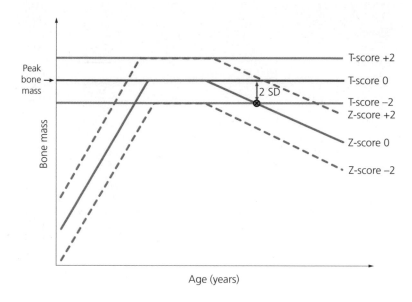

Figure 4.1 The derivation of T- and Z-scores. The point marked by a cross demonstrates a bone mass value lying 2 standard deviations (SD) below the mean reference value for premenopausal women (peak bone mass) and therefore illustrates a T-score of –2. The dotted lines indicate Z-scores of +2 and –2.

Dual-energy X-ray absorptiometry (DXA) is widely regarded as the diagnostic method of choice. In this test, differential absorption of two X-ray frequencies by soft tissue and bone enables bone mass to be calculated (Figures 4.2–4.4). DXA is applied to both the axial and appendicular skeleton; the most commonly assessed sites are the femoral neck, lumbar spine and radius. The measurements can take as little as 1–2 minutes and are achieved at a very low dose of radiation. The patient is simply required to lie on the couch during the measurements, with the hips and knees flexed to straighten the lumbar spine (see Figure 4.2a).

The newest absorptiometry systems also have the potential to generate high-quality lateral images of the thoracic and lumbar spine (see Figure 4.2b).

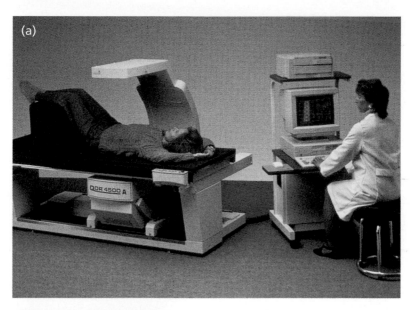

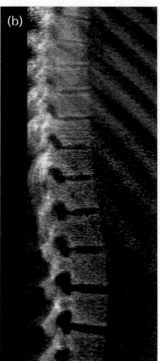

Figure 4.2 The dual-energy X-ray absorptiometry system. (a) The patient lies on the couch with hips and knees flexed to straighten the lumbar spine while measurements are taken. (b) A lateral image of the spine obtained using a Hologic QDR-4500 absorptiometer.

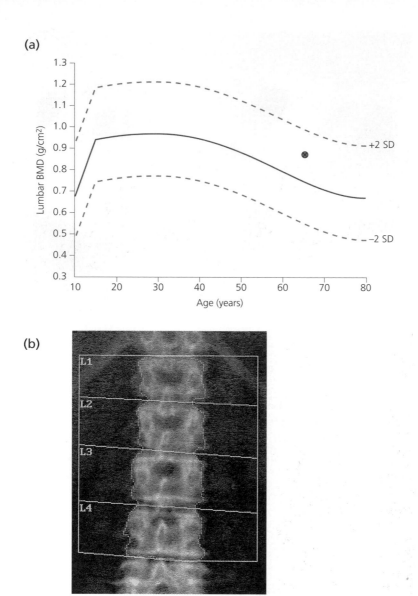

Figure 4.3 Printout of a lumbar spine measurement by dual-energy X-ray absorptiometry. (a) The value for the patient's bone mineral density (BMD), shown by the cross, is plotted in relation to reference data. (b) The image of the lumbar spine (L1–L4) is also shown. SD, standard deviation.

(a)

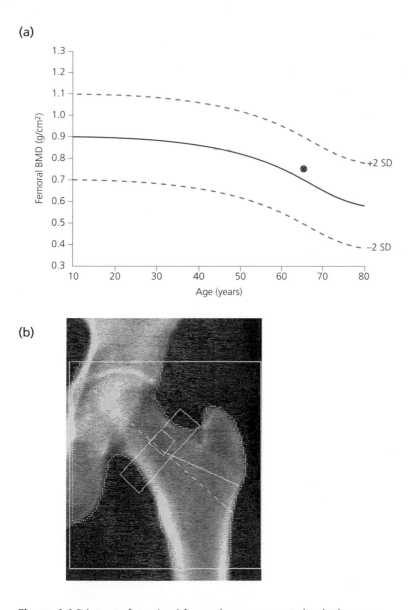

(b)

Figure 4.4 Printout of proximal femoral measurements by dual-energy X-ray absorptiometry. (a) The value for bone mineral density (BMD), shown by the cross, is plotted in relation to reference data. (b) The image of the proximal femur on which sites of measurement are shown. SD, standard deviation.

Semiautomated analyses can be performed on these images to assess vertebral deformity at a fraction of the radiation dose required for conventional spinal radiography.

Spinal measurements made by DXA may be inaccurate in the presence of osteophytes, extraskeletal calcification, vertebral fracture or spinal deformity (e.g. scoliosis). As all of these conditions are relatively common in the elderly, the usefulness of spinal measurements in this age group is limited.

Quantitative computed tomography, although available in a few centers only, can be used to measure bone mass in both the axial and appendicular skeleton. The radiation dose is significantly higher than for DXA.

Quantitative ultrasound (QUS) measures broadband attenuation and speed of sound at various skeletal sites. Most investigators now believe that QUS of the calcaneus yields a quantitative measurement of bone mass similar to, although not the same as, the bone density measurement obtained by DXA. Claims that ultrasound provides a measure of bone 'quality' have not been substantiated.

Most commonly, QUS measurements are taken of the calcaneus because it is easily accessible, has a high (> 90%) trabecular bone content, is responsive to gravitational forces and is relatively small in size. In addition, portability, low cost and lack of ionizing radiation have made this mode of imaging popular for mass screening. Furthermore, prospective studies of postmenopausal women have demonstrated that QUS of the calcaneus is predictive of fracture risk: a QUS measurement 1 SD below young normal is associated with approximately double the risk of hip fracture. In general, stiffness or stiffness index, a mathematical term derived from speed of sound and broadband attenuation, is provided as a raw score, together with an estimated BMD and a T-score.

However, even when used at the same anatomic site, different QUS machines and distinct normative databases can lead to confusion in defining risk from a manufacturer-specific T-score, particularly when it is related to the criteria defined by the World Health Organization (see Table 4.2, page 33).

Notwithstanding these issues, precision has improved considerably, and allows for repeated measurements over time; an error of approximately 2% at the calcaneus is now noted for most machines. However, the use of QUS in monitoring therapy has not been validated.

Newer technologies include scanning devices to assess multiple bones, and finger DXA and ultrasounds. Multiple site determinations enhance the likelihood of demonstrating low bone mass in at least one skeletal site.

Fracture detection

Conventional radiography is an insensitive method for assessing bone loss but plays a major role in the diagnosis of fracture. Diagnosis of fractures of the wrist, hip, pelvis and long bones is relatively straightforward.

The definition and diagnosis of vertebral fracture is, however, more difficult because:

- the majority of vertebral fractures are relatively asymptomatic and do not come to medical attention
- vertebral shape between and within individuals varies, leading to uncertainty about the degree of change that signifies a clinically significant pathological event.

Three types of vertebral fracture may occur: biconcave, wedge, and compression or crush (see Figure 3.1, page 26; Figure 4.5). In clinical practice, a change that is obvious on visual inspection is likely to be significant, but the importance of lesser degrees of deformity is often more difficult to assess. Other conditions that may result in vertebral fracture (e.g. epiphysitis and osteoarthritis) should be excluded.

The presence of radiological osteopenia may indicate low bone mass. Although this is a purely qualitative assessment, and technical factors, such as exposure, influence the radiodensity of bone, unequivocal osteopenia is usually a sign of advanced bone loss.

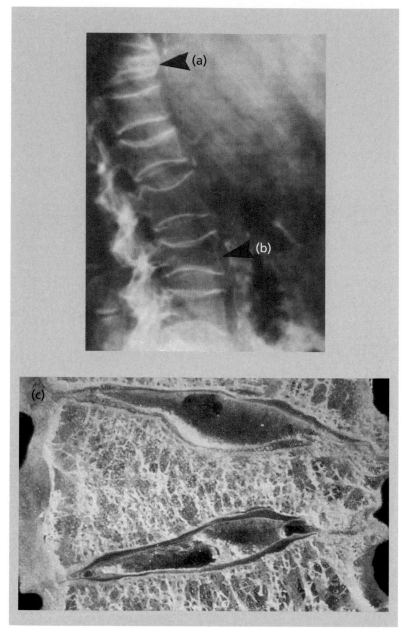

Figure 4.5 Three types of vertebral deformity occur: (a) compression fracture (arrow); (b) biconcavity of lower vertebrae (arrow); (c) wedge fracture.

TABLE 4.3
Biochemical markers of bone turnover

Resorption
- N-terminal and C-terminal cross-linked telopeptides of type 1 collagen (NTx, CTX)
- Urinary deoxypyridinoline and pyridinoline
- Serum tartrate-resistant acid phosphatase

Formation
- Serum bone-specific alkaline phosphatase
- Serum osteocalcin
- Serum type-1 procollagen peptides (e.g. P1NP)

Biochemical markers of bone turnover

A number of products of collagen breakdown or of bone cells that reflect bone turnover have been identified (Table 4.3). These biochemical markers provide information about the rate of bone loss at the time of measurement.

Although the wide variation in levels of markers within and between individuals makes them unsuitable as primary diagnostic tools, they do show significant reductions during antiresorptive therapy and may be helpful in determining responsiveness to treatment. However, at present, their use is mainly restricted to research applications.

Two prospective studies in older individuals suggest that resorption markers may be useful in identifying those at high risk of hip fracture, supporting the tenet that qualitative changes in bone are important determinants of subsequent fracture risk.

Differential diagnosis

A number of diseases are associated with osteoporosis (Table 4.4). Secondary disorders are present in around 40% of osteoporotic men, but are much less common in women. In some cases, the diagnosis may be evident on clinical examination, but common secondary causes should be excluded in all patients presenting with osteoporosis.

TABLE 4.4

Secondary causes of osteoporosis

Endocrine disorders

- Primary and secondary hypogonadism
- Thyrotoxicosis
- Hyperparathyroidism
- Cushing's syndrome
- Hyperprolactinemia

Malignant disease

- Myelomatosis
- Leukemia
- Lymphoma
- Mastocytosis

Connective tissue disorders

- Osteogenesis imperfecta
- Marfan's syndrome
- Ehlers–Danlos syndrome
- Homocystinuria

Drugs

- Alcohol
- Glucocorticoids
- Heparin
- Aromatase inhibitors (used to treat breast cancer)
- Gonadotropin-releasing hormone analogs (used to treat prostate cancer)
- Selective serotonin-receptor reuptake inhibitors
- Thiazolidenediones
- Proton pump inhibitors

Other causes

- Malabsorption/bowel disease
- Gastrectomy
- Chronic liver disease
- Chronic obstructive pulmonary disease
- Chronic renal disease
- Transplantation
- Rheumatoid arthritis
- Immobilization

Routine investigations to exclude secondary causes of osteoporosis should include:

- a complete blood count and measurement of erythrocyte sedimentation rate
- measurement of serum calcium, phosphate and alkaline phosphatase

- measurement of serum parathyroid hormone, if hypercalcemia is present
- liver function tests
- thyroid function tests
- serum protein immunoelectrophoresis
- measurement of urinary Bence-Jones proteins
- measurement of endomysial and/or tissue transglutaminase antibodies for celiac disease.

If they have not already been performed, lateral radiographs of the thoracic and lumbar spine should be obtained to check for vertebral deformity. Other investigations may be indicated if there is a high index of clinical suspicion and/or abnormalities are revealed by routine tests. It should also be noted that in a few cases of myeloma, serum and urinary proteins may be normal, and bone marrow trephine is required to establish the diagnosis. Isotopic bone scanning is useful in cases of suspected malignancy, and bone biopsy may be required to confirm the diagnosis in osteomalacia.

Key points – diagnostic techniques

- A careful history and examination should be performed in all patients suspected of having osteoporosis, including examination for secondary causes of osteoporosis in women as well as men.
- Diagnostic classification is based on T-scores (standard deviations derived from reference data from premenopausal women).
- Dual-energy X-ray absorptiometry (DXA) is widely regarded as the diagnostic method of choice, although spinal measurements may be inaccurate, particularly in the elderly.
- Diagnosis of vertebral fractures requires lateral thoracic spine and lumbar spine images, using either conventional X-rays or DXA.
- Biochemical markers of bone turnover are mainly restricted to research applications, but may prove useful in determining response to treatment.

In men with osteoporosis, a more thorough investigation is required. Hypogonadism is a common secondary cause, and measurement of serum testosterone and gonadotropins should be routine. In patients with low testosterone but normal gonadotropin levels, serum prolactin should be assessed.

It is important to note that alcohol abuse and glucocorticoid treatment are relatively common causes of secondary osteoporosis in men.

Key references

Binkley N, Krueger D, Gangnon R et al. Lateral vertebral assessment: a valuable technique to detect clinically significant vertebral fractures. *Osteoporos Int* 2005;16:1513–8.

Genant HK, Engelke K, Prevrhal S. Advanced CT bone imaging in osteoporosis. *Rheumatology (Oxford)* 2008;47 (suppl 4):9–16.

Seibel MJ. Biochemical markers of bone metabolism in the assessment of osteoporosis: useful or not? *J Endocrinol Invest* 2003;26:464–71.

Siris E, Brenneman SK, Barrett-Connor E et al. The effect of age and bone mineral density on the absolute, excess, and relative risk of fracture in postmenopausal women aged 50-99: results from the National Osteoporosis Risk Assessment (NORA). *Osteoporos Int* 2006; 17:565–74.

Bone mineral density and clinical risk factors: the WHO paradigm

In clinical practice, bone mineral density (BMD) values are used to predict fracture risk, in much the same way that blood pressure is used to predict stroke. Prospective studies in postmenopausal women have shown that for each decrease of 1 standard deviation in BMD, there is a two- to three-fold increase in fracture risk (Figure 5.1). The strength of this association is comparable with that between blood pressure and stroke, or serum lipid profile and coronary heart disease. Measurements at the potential fracture site are the most predictive, although bone density at the wrist, spine, calcaneus or hip is related to fracture risk at any skeletal site.

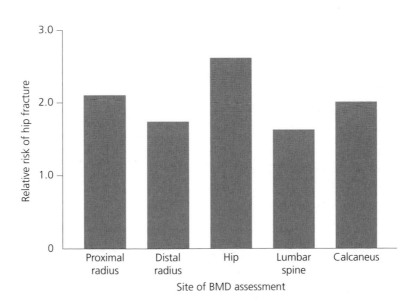

Figure 5.1 Relative risk of hip fracture for every 1 standard deviation (SD) reduction in bone mineral density (BMD) below the age-adjusted mean. Adapted from data in Marshall D et al. *BMJ* 1996;312:1254–9.

BMD measurements have a high specificity but low sensitivity in the prediction of fracture risk, and recent studies have demonstrated that the majority of fractures occur in individuals with osteopenia rather than osteoporosis. This is partly due to the contribution of clinical risk factors that affect fracture risk independently of BMD, and these can be used to improve prediction of fracture risk. They include:

- age
- body mass index ≤ 19 kg/m^2
- glucocorticoid therapy
- previous history of fracture
- family history of hip fracture
- current smoking
- alcohol ≥ 3 units/day
- rheumatoid arthritis.

A World Health Organization-supported algorithm that combines these risk factors with or without BMD measurements to estimate fracture probability has been developed recently, and is available online at www.shef.ac.uk/FRAX (Figure 5.2). This simple and rapid-to-use tool produces estimates of the 10-year probability of major osteoporotic fracture (hip, spine, humerus and radius) and hip fracture alone.

These figures can then be used as a basis for treatment decisions, taking into account cost-effectiveness and clinical effectiveness (Figure 5.3).

Guidelines using this approach have been developed in Europe and the USA.

The FRAX® estimation of fracture probability takes no account of previous bone-protective treatment or of dose responses for several risk factors. For example, multiple fractures carry a much higher risk than a single fracture, and the increase in risk of fracture with glucocorticoid therapy is related to both dose and duration of therapy. These limitations emphasize the need for clinical judgment when using FRAX® as a basis for treatment decisions.

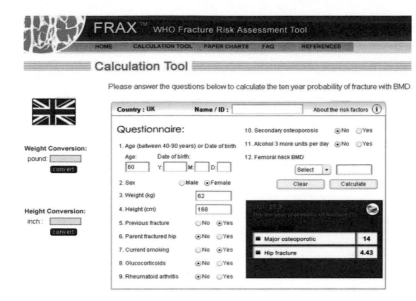

Figure 5.2 The FRAX® tool: 10-year fracture probability is estimated from the data input, with or without bone mineral density measurement. Note that both the 10-year probability of major osteoporotic fracture (spine, hip, wrist, humerus), at 14%, and hip fracture, at 4.4%, are estimated. Reproduced with permission of the World Health Organization Collaborating Centre for Metabolic Bone Diseases, University of Sheffield Medical School, UK. www.shef.ac.uk/FRAX.

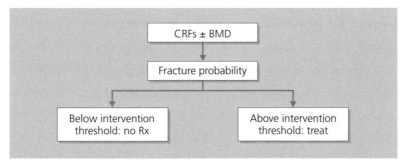

Figure 5.3 Paradigm for risk assessment and treatment decisions. On the basis of clinical risk factors (CRF), with or without bone mineral density (BMD) measurement, the 10-year fracture probability is estimated and used as a basis for management decisions. Intervention thresholds are defined on the basis of both cost-effectiveness and clinical suitability.

47

Other risk factors

Other risk factors for osteoporosis (see Table 2.1, page 18 and
Table 4.4, page 42), increase fracture risk by reducing BMD
and include:

- untreated premature menopause
- hypogonadism
- endocrine disease
- gastrointestinal disease
- organ transplantation
- chronic obstructive pulmonary disease
- immobility
- dietary problems (e.g. low calcium intake, high caffeine intake)
- vitamin D insufficiency.

Identification of these risk factors is clinically important because
many of them can be modified.

The risk of falling is a major determinant of fracture, particularly for
hip fracture in the elderly. Factors that increase the likelihood of falls
include environmental hazards, medication and health problems,
particularly neurological disorders (Table 5.1). Some of these risk
factors are modifiable.

TABLE 5.1

Factors that increase the risk of falling

Environmental

- Uneven paving stones,
  steps, loose carpets, etc.

Health-related

- Poor cognitive function
  (e.g. dementia)
- Poor visual acuity
- Physical disability
- Neuromuscular dysfunction

Drugs

- Alcohol
- Benzodiazepines
- Anticonvulsants

Who should undergo risk assessment?

At present there is no universal agreement that population-based screening to identify individuals at high risk from fracture can be justified. Current practice is to use a case-finding strategy in which individuals with risk factors undergo further assessment. These may be either risk factors used in the FRAX algorithm or those risk factors that mediate their effect through reducing BMD.

Because age is a major determinant of fracture risk (Figure 5.4), case finding is mainly restricted to postmenopausal women and men aged over 50 years. Absolute fracture risk is very low in the majority of younger people, even with low BMD, and hence bone protective therapy is rarely indicated. It should be noted that FRAX is only appropriate as

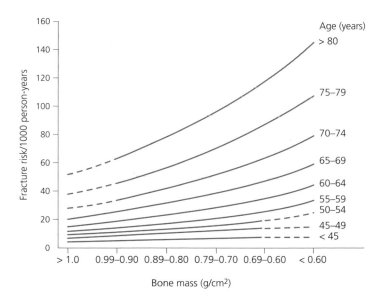

Figure 5.4 Estimated incidence of non-spinal fractures in relation to age and bone mass in 521 white women followed up for an average of 6.5 years. Bone mass was measured in the midshaft of the radius. Republished from Hui SL et al. *J Clin Invest* 1988;81:1804–9. Reproduced with permission of the American Society for Clinical Investigation, © 1988, via the Copyright Clearance Center.

a risk assessment tool for postmenopausal women and older men. In younger men and women, there is very little evidence on which to base fracture risk assessment, either from clinical risk factors or bone densitometry.

In some cases, clinical risk factors alone are sufficient to make a treatment decision and BMD measurement is not required. For example, an 80-year-old woman with multiple fragility fractures can normally be referred for treatment without further investigation, provided that other causes of fracture have been excluded.

Key points – risk assessment

- Bone mineral density (BMD) is inversely related to fracture risk and can be used to predict fracture risk.
- Addition of clinical risk factors for fracture that are independent of BMD improve the prediction of fracture.
- The FRAX™ risk assessment tool, supported by the World Health Organization, provides a simple and rapid means of estimating 10-year fracture probability, on which intervention thresholds can be based.
- At present, a case-finding strategy is recommended to identify individuals at high risk of fracture, based on clinical risk factors.

Key references

Greenspan SL, Myers ER, Kiel DP et al. Fall direction, bone mineral density, and function: risk factors for hip fracture in frail nursing home elderly. Am J Med 1998;104:539–45.

Kanis JA, Burlet N, Cooper C et al. European guidance for the diagnosis and management of osteoporosis in postmenopausal women. Osteoporos Int 2008;19:399–428 [Erratum in Osteoporos Int 2008;19:1103–4].

Kanis JA, Johnell O, Oden A et al. Ten-year risk of osteoporotic fracture and the effect of risk factors on screening strategies. Bone 2002; 30:251–8.

Kanis JA, Oden A, Johnell et al. The use of clinical risk factors enhances the performance of BMD in the prediction of hip and osteoporotic fractures in men and women. Osteoporos Int 2007;18:1033–46.

National Osteoporosis Society. Position statements on bone densitometry (include quantitative ultrasound, peripheral and central dual-energy X-ray absorptiometry, provision of a bone densitometry service). www.nos.org.uk

Siris E, Delmas PD. Assessment of 10-year absolute fracture risk: a new paradigm with worldwide application. *Osteoporos Int* 2008;19:383–4.

Tosteson AN, Melton LJ 3rd, Dawson-Hughes B et al. Cost-effective osteoporosis treatment thresholds: the United States perspective. *Osteoporos Int* 2008;19:437–47.

van Helden S, van Geel AC, Geusens PP et al. Bone and fall-related fracture risks in women and men with a recent clinical fracture. *J Bone Joint Surg Am* 2008;90: 241–8.

Factors affecting the choice of intervention

Since fragility fractures are the only clinical consequence of
osteoporosis, the main aim of treatment is to reduce the risk
of fracture and to alleviate the symptoms associated with fracture.

A number of pharmacological agents have been shown to reduce
the risk of fracture in randomized controlled trials. Most of these studies
have been conducted in postmenopausal women with osteoporosis or
established osteoporosis, although in the case of hormone replacement
therapy (HRT) fracture reduction was demonstrated in healthy
postmenopausal women.

Many studies have also demonstrated the efficacy of these drugs in
terms of bone density or changes in bone turnover. In clinical practice,
a positive change in bone mineral density (BMD) or suppression of
bone resorption have been considered reasonable endpoints for
providers and patients. However, there is often a disparity between
the change in bone mass and fracture risk reduction, such that very
modest improvements, or even no change from baseline, is associated
with fracture risk reduction.

In addition, changes in bone turnover markers are often difficult
to interpret due to patient variability. Hence, the choice of intervention
and the parameters used to follow up patients depend on a number
of factors.

Protection against fractures. Fracture reduction has not been assessed
in head-to-head trials between different agents, so it is not possible to
compare the efficacy of these agents directly. However, some, but not
all, interventions have been shown to protect against vertebral and non-
vertebral (particularly hip) fractures (Table 6.1). This is an important
distinction, because once a fragility fracture has occurred, the risk of
fracture at that site and elsewhere is increased; ideally, a treatment
should protect against fractures at all common sites, especially the
spine and hip. There is evidence for such protection in the case of

TABLE 6.1

Efficacy of pharmacological interventions for osteoporosis on vertebral, non-vertebral and hip fractures. Note that alendronate, risedronate, HRT, strontium ranelate and zoledronate have all been shown to reduce fractures at all three sites.

Intervention	Vertebral	Non-vertebral	Hip
Alendronate	+	+	+
Risedronate	+	+	+
Ibandronate	+	+†	Nae
Etidronate	+	Nae	Nae
HRT	+	+	+
Raloxifene	+	Nae	Nae
Calcitriol	+*	Nae	Nae
Calcitonin	+*	Nae	Nae
Teriparatide	+	+	Nae
PTH (1-84)	+	Nae	Nae
Strontium ranelate	+	+	+†
Zoledronate	+	+	+

+, Positive effect: reduces fractures; Nae, not adequately evaluated.
*Inconsistent data.
†Demonstrated in post-hoc analysis.
HRT, hormone replacement therapy; PTH, parathyroid hormone.

alendronate, risedronate, zoledronate and strontium ranelate in postmenopausal women with osteoporosis, and for HRT in healthy postmenopausal women.

Safety and tolerability are important issues in the positioning of treatments for osteoporosis. Since treatment is given over the long term (usually for at least 5 years), is not associated with symptomatic improvement and may cause side effects, it is essential that patient preference is carefully considered before deciding on a particular treatment option. Intermittent regimens may have an advantage in this respect for many women.

Extraskeletal risks and benefits are potentially important when prescribing HRT or raloxifene, and these considerations are discussed in more detail in the following chapters. However, recent evidence indicating that the risk–benefit profile of HRT may be less favorable than was previously believed has led to a reduction in its use in the treatment of osteoporosis.

Cost-effectiveness is an increasingly important consideration when choosing a therapy. Recent analyses of the cost-effectiveness of different interventions indicate that bisphosphonates, strontium ranelate and raloxifene are cost-effective in postmenopausal women with established osteoporosis and in those without fracture but with a high fracture probability.

Mechanisms of action

Bone resorption. Until recently, drugs used in the treatment of osteoporosis were predominantly antiresorptive, that is, they acted by inhibiting bone resorption. These drugs, which include the bisphosphonates, raloxifene, HRT, calcitriol and calcitonin, mainly act to prevent menopausal and age-related bone loss.

The use of antiresorptive drugs is associated with an initial increase in BMD as a result of 'catch-up' bone formation (Figure 6.1), followed by either a plateau or, in the case of more potent antiresorptive agents such as alendronate, a sustained although smaller increase in BMD due to increased secondary mineralization of bone.

Bone formation. Anabolic agents such as parathyroid hormone (PTH) peptides and sodium fluoride act by increasing bone formation. The use of these agents is associated with a larger and sustained increase in BMD (Figure 6.2).

Other mechanisms of action. Evidence indicates that strontium ranelate acts differently from other bone-protective interventions, strengthening bone by a mechanism believed to involve changes in the bone matrix/mineral composite while maintaining bone formation in association with reduced resorption.

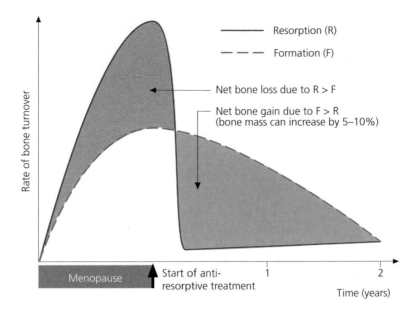

Figure 6.1 Bone turnover is the key to understanding treatment for osteoporosis. Although both bone resorption and bone formation accelerate during menopause, resorption outstrips formation. Antiresorptive therapy (arrow) blocks resorption, thereby allowing formation to 'catch up' with resorption. During this catch-up phase, the transient formation may actually exceed resorption for a short period. Eventually bone mass reaches a plateau. If the imbalance between resorption and formation remains then bone loss will resume, as resorption again exceeds formation.

Response to treatment

Although in the untreated state BMD is a strong predictor of fracture risk, the magnitude of increase in BMD induced by intervention is a poor predictor of antifracture efficacy. In contrast, there is some evidence that reduction in biochemical markers of resorption after treatment with antiresorptive drugs may predict fracture reduction, emphasizing the importance of bone turnover as a determinant of bone strength. The role of bone markers in predicting response to PTH peptide and strontium ranelate is less clear.

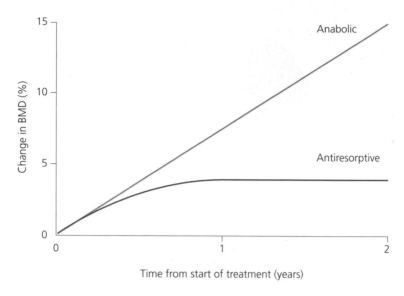

Figure 6.2 Potential changes in bone mineral density (BMD) due to either antiresorptive therapy or stimulation of bone formation by anabolic agents.

Treatment has a relatively rapid effect on fracture, with significant reductions seen within 6–18 months. The rate at which these effects wear off when treatment is stopped is less certain. In general, bone loss resumes within a year or so, although there may be longer-lasting effects with potent bisphosphonates such as alendronate. The optimal duration of treatment is unclear. On the one hand, resumption of bone loss after withdrawal of therapy could be associated with increased fracture risk, suggesting that treatment should be indefinite. On the other hand, there are potential concerns that long-term suppression of bone turnover with antiresorptive agents may increase microdamage and reduce bone strength.

Non-pharmacological interventions

In addition to measures that reduce fracture risk, management of the patient with osteoporosis should include:

- lifestyle advice
- symptomatic treatment
- psychological and social support.

The risk of falling should be carefully assessed and modifiable risk factors must be addressed. Hip protectors, which reduce the impact of falling on the femoral neck and trochanter, are probably effective in institutionalized individuals, but their use is limited by poor compliance.

Lifestyle advice includes advice about dietary calcium intake and vitamin D status, avoidance of tobacco use and alcohol abuse, and appropriate levels of physical activity.

Physical activity. Loss of the effect of gravity on the skeleton (e.g. immobilization) produces a dramatic reduction in bone mass due to uncoupling of the bone remodeling unit. Bone resorption increases dramatically while bone formation is markedly suppressed. Evidence that exercise can have a positive impact on BMD in older patients is less compelling than data from studies in younger individuals. However, several trials do suggest that, like calcium, weight-bearing exercise can slow or prevent further bone loss. The mechanisms responsible for this effect have not been well defined but, in one study at least, calcium supplementation plus regular exercise provided better protection against femoral bone loss in older postmenopausal women than placebo or calcium supplementation alone. In addition, maintaining adequate levels of physical activity in older people may reduce the risk of falls and improve the protective neuromuscular responses to falling. Therefore, regular weight-bearing exercise is another important component in the management of osteoporosis.

The degree of exercise should be tailored to the individual, but brisk walking for 30 minutes on 3–4 days each week should be undertaken when possible. In frail elderly people, more gentle exercises such as tai chi are useful in maintaining muscle tone and balance, and may reduce the risk of falls.

Symptomatic treatment. Analgesia should be prescribed when necessary for pain relief. Physiotherapy is also often helpful in reducing pain, improving posture and muscle strength, and rebuilding confidence.

Psychological and social support. Support groups are helpful for many sufferers and their carers in providing information, practical advice and psychological support. A list of such organizations is provided on pages 96–7 of this book.

Monitoring of treatment

In most patients with osteoporosis, bone densitometry is the only way to assess long-term response to treatment, and the procedure may be used to reassure a patient that the treatment is effective and hence improve compliance. The ability of bone densitometry to reflect actual treatment effects depends on the precision of the measurement technique, the expected rate of bone loss in the absence of treatment and the magnitude of the change induced by treatment. In general, demonstration of a significant treatment effect in an individual patient requires approximately 2 years for the spine and at least 3 years for the hip; thus, identification of non-responders by this means is far from ideal. Furthermore, the percentage of true non-responders is believed to be low, so that in most cases regular monitoring of treatment is unlikely to alter patient management. A more rational approach is to measure BMD at the end of the proposed treatment period (usually 5–10 years) to assess whether further intervention is required to protect the skeleton.

Most cases of non-response are due to poor compliance and persistence. They can be improved by careful explanation of the need for treatment, discussion of possible side effects and reassurance about the well-documented effect of interventions on fracture risk (but not symptoms). In addition, studies have shown that contact with a health professional a few months after starting treatment to reinforce this advice improves compliance and persistence.

Monitoring by bone densitometry is recommended in situations in which response to therapy is less predictable, for example in patients receiving high doses of glucocorticoids or those with malabsorption, and in patient groups in whom the effects of treatment are not well documented, such as men and premenopausal women.

Measurement of biochemical markers may also be used to monitor treatment. However, the biological variability of these markers and measurement variance limit this application in individual patients and, as yet, there is no robust evidence that this approach improves outcomes.

Key points – management: general considerations

- Treatment for osteoporosis is aimed at reducing fracture risk and alleviating symptoms related to fracture.
- Available pharmacological interventions include alendronate, ibandronate, risedronate, zoledronate, raloxifene, strontium ranelate, teriparatide, parathyroid hormone peptides and hormone replacement therapy.
- Patient preference is an important factor in determining treatment choice.
- Drugs may reduce fracture risk by inhibiting bone resorption, increasing bone formation or a combination of the two.
- Non-pharmacological approaches include lifestyle advice, physiotherapy and (in institutionalized elderly individuals) hip protectors.
- In general, regular monitoring of treatment is unlikely to alter patient management, but bone densitometry is recommended if the response to therapy is likely to be unpredictable (e.g. in men, premenopausal women and patients receiving high-dose glucocorticoids).

Key references

Delmas PD. Different effects of antiresorptive therapies on vertebral and nonvertebral fractures in postmenopausal osteoporosis. *Bone* 2002;30:14–17.

Feder G, Cryer C, Donovan S, Carter Y. Guidelines for the prevention of falls in people over 65. The Guidelines' Development Group. *BMJ* 2000;321:1007–11.

Kanis JA, Adams J, Borgström F et al. The cost-effectiveness of alendronate in the management of osteoporosis. *Bone* 2008;42:4–15.

Kannus P, Parkkari J, Khan K. Hip protectors need an evidence base. *Lancet* 2003;362:1168–9.

Bisphosphonates

The bisphosphonates have a basic pyrophosphate structure and inhibit bone resorption. The ability of bisphosphonates to reach bone directly with almost no extraskeletal side effects, yet increase bone mass and reduce both vertebral and hip fractures when administered properly, has resulted in wide use of these agents. As all the bisphosphonates have very poor bioavailability and bind calcium avidly, etidronate, alendronate, risedronate and the oral formulation of ibandronate are taken on an empty stomach with water only. Alternatively, intravenous formulations of ibandronate and zoledronate are now available. Bisphosphonates are considered a first-line treatment for osteoporosis. In addition, some are licensed for the treatment of metastatic bone disease, and some are being investigated for the prevention of malignancy-associated bone disease in myeloma and breast cancer (see Chapter 2, Pathophysiology).

Alendronate. Oral alendronate is one of the second-generation bisphosphonates, a drug class that has enjoyed greater use in the last decade. Alendronate does not impair mineralization, but is a potent antiresorptive agent, and is widely used to treat women with osteoporosis.

Efficacy. In the vertebral fracture arm of the Fracture Intervention Trial (FIT, a study of approximately 2000 women with existing vertebral fracture), daily administration of alendronate for 3 years halved the risk of a new vertebral fracture and reduced the risk of having two or more vertebral fractures by 90%. Furthermore, the risk of having a hip or wrist fracture declined by approximately 50% (Figure 7.1). These decreases in fracture risk were associated with a rise in bone density of 3.2% in the hip and 8% in the lumbar spine. Furthermore, symptomatic spine fractures were diminished by nearly 60% after 12 months and the presence of any symptomatic fracture was reduced by 27% after 18 months. Pooled data from all published

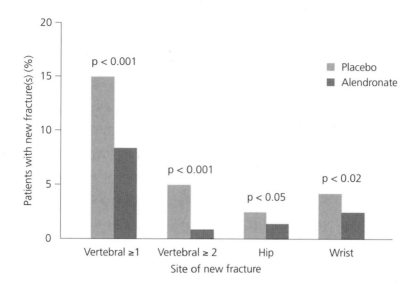

Figure 7.1 Significant reductions in the risk of new fractures in the spine, hip and wrist have been demonstrated in alendronate-treated patients. The figure shows the percentage of patients suffering a new fracture after 3 years of treatment with oral alendronate or placebo in a randomized controlled, double-blind study in women with existing vertebral fracture. Adapted from data in Black DM et al. 1996.

treatment and prevention trials of alendronate reveal a reduction of approximately 30% for any clinical fracture and of almost 50% for new morphometric vertebral fractures (radiographic evidence).

In the other arm of FIT (variously called FIT II or the clinical fracture arm of FIT), in women with a femoral-neck bone mineral density (BMD) T-score below –1.6, with or without prevalent vertebral fractures, alendronate reduced the risk of new morphometric vertebral fractures by 44%. In women with T-scores of –2.5 or less, there was a 56% reduction in the risk of hip fractures and a 36% reduction in the risk of all clinical fractures.

In summary, alendronate treatment for women with established osteoporosis results in a fairly rapid and significant reduction in both spine and non-vertebral fractures. Women who benefit most from alendronate treatment are those at high risk, for example women over

65 years of age with previous fractures and very low bone mass. Although there is also a consistent increase in BMD with alendronate, it is clear that not all of the reduction in fracture risk can be attributed purely to the change in BMD. Reduction in bone turnover, preservation of skeletal architecture and increased mineralization of bone may also contribute to the strong antifracture efficacy of alendronate and the other bisphosphonates.

Tolerability. In clinical trials of over 6000 women, the frequency of adverse upper gastrointestinal effects was not increased in those taking alendronate versus placebo. However, since the drug's release severe erosive esophagitis has been described in a few patients, and alendronate should therefore be avoided in patients who have abnormalities of the esophagus. To minimize the risk of esophagitis, patients should be instructed to swallow the tablet with a full glass of plain water on an empty stomach at least 30 minutes before breakfast (and any other oral medication), to stand or sit upright for at least 30 minutes, and not to lie down after eating breakfast. The tablets should not be taken at bedtime or before rising.

Dose and indication. Alendronate is licensed for prevention and treatment of postmenopausal osteoporosis as a once-daily (5 mg or 10 mg) or once-weekly (35 mg or 70 mg) formulation. The recommended dose in postmenopausal women not receiving hormone replacement therapy (HRT) is 10 mg daily or 70 mg weekly. Effects on BMD with the once-weekly formulations are similar to those observed with a daily dose of 10 mg, though no fracture data are available. Alendronate is also approved for the treatment of men with osteoporosis (10 mg daily), and for the prevention and treatment of glucocorticoid-induced osteoporosis (5 mg daily).

Risedronate, another second-generation, nitrogen-containing bisphosphonate, is also approved for use in Europe and the USA for the treatment of both men and women with osteoporosis.

Efficacy. In two large, multicenter trials (in Europe and North America), more than 3600 postmenopausal women, all of whom had at least one vertebral fracture, received risedronate, 5 mg or 2.5 mg daily. The 2.5 mg formulation was dropped, but 5 mg dosing was continued throughout the study, and after 3 years there was almost a 45% reduction in new vertebral fractures and a statistically significant reduction in non-vertebral fractures (except hip fractures). There was no reduction in new hip fractures, but there was an increase in spine BMD of approximately 5% and hip BMD of 3% compared with placebo results. The antifracture efficacy was evident as early as 1 year after the start of therapy (Figure 7.2).

Reduction in hip fracture with risedronate treatment has also been demonstrated in a large, randomized controlled trial. Two groups of postmenopausal women were studied: 5445 (aged 70–79 years) with

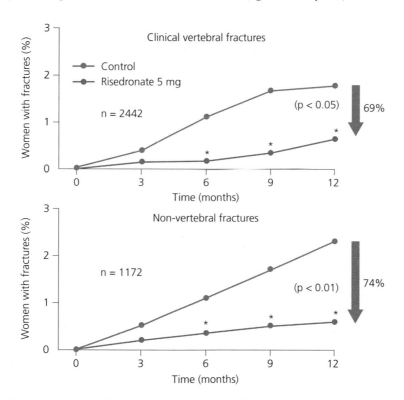

Figure 7.2 Onset of fracture risk reduction: effect of risedronate in postmenopausal women with osteoporosis. *Statistically significant difference from control. Reproduced with permission from Roux et al. *Curr Med Res Opin* 2004;20:433–9 and Harrington et al. *Calcif Tissue Int* 2004;74:129–35.

osteoporosis of the hip and at least one risk factor for falling, and 3886 (aged ≥ 80 years) who had either osteoporosis of the hip or at least one risk factor for falling. Overall, the incidence of hip fracture in women treated with risedronate, 2.5 mg or 5 mg daily, was 2.8% compared with 3.9% in the control group (relative risk [RR] 0.7; 95% confidence interval [CI] 0.6–0.9). When the two groups were analyzed separately, a significant reduction in hip fracture was seen in the younger group with osteoporosis of the hip (RR 0.6; 95% CI 0.4–0.9) but there was no significant reduction in the group of women aged 80 years or over.

In a 2-year trial of 284 men with osteoporosis, risedronate, 35 mg once weekly, produced significant improvements in lumbar spine BMD at 6, 12 and 24 months.

Tolerability. In clinical trials, risedronate was not associated with any increase in upper gastrointestinal adverse effects despite the inclusion of women with risk factors for, or with existing, upper gastrointestinal disease. Nevertheless, it is important, as with alendronate, that patients are instructed to swallow the tablet with a full glass of plain water on an empty stomach in an upright position, and to stand or sit for at least 30 minutes afterwards. The tablet can be taken at any time of day, but food and drink must be avoided for at least 2 hours before or after taking it.

Dose and indication. Risedronate is available as a once-daily (5 mg), once-weekly (35 mg) or once-monthly (150 mg) formulation for the prevention of osteoporosis and for the treatment of postmenopausal osteoporosis to reduce the risk of vertebral or hip fractures. Risedronate, 5 mg daily, is approved for the treatment of osteoporosis in men and for the prevention and treatment of glucocorticoid-induced osteoporosis in postmenopausal women.

Ibandronate is also a nitrogen-containing bisphosphonate, and is approved for osteoporosis in Europe and the USA.

Efficacy. The effects of two oral regimens of ibandronate on vertebral fracture in postmenopausal women with osteoporosis were examined in the BONE study (oral iBandronate Osteoporosis vertebral fracture trial in North America and Europe). In total, 2946 women were randomized to receive either placebo, daily ibandronate

(2.5 mg/day) or intermittent ibandronate (20 mg on alternate days for
12 doses every 3 months). After 3 years of treatment the rate of new
vertebral fractures was reduced by 62% and 50% with daily and
intermittent ibandronate, respectively, relative to placebo (Figure 7.3).
Increases in lumbar spine and total hip BMD of around 5% and
3.5–4.0%, respectively, relative to placebo, were seen in ibandronate-
treated women. No reduction in non-vertebral fractures was
demonstrated in the intention-to-treat analysis, although a post hoc
analysis in a subgroup showed a reduction in non-vertebral fractures
in the daily but not in the intermittent treatment group.

Subsequently, the effects of other oral regimens of ibandronate on
BMD in postmenopausal women with osteoporosis have been reported.
In the MOBILE (Monthly Oral iBandronate In LadiEs) study,

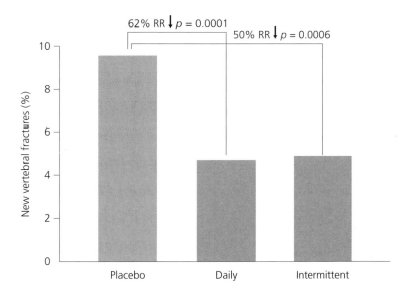

Figure 7.3 Effect of 3 years of treatment with two regimens of oral
ibandronate on the incidence of vertebral fractures in postmenopausal
women with osteoporosis. Patients were randomized to a daily regimen
(2.5 mg/day) or an intermittent regimen (20 mg on alternate days for
12 doses every 3 months). Reproduced from Chesnut et al. 2004, with
permission of the American Society for Bone and Mineral Research.
Copyright © 2004.

1609 women were randomized to receive 2.5 mg daily, 50 mg + 50 mg monthly (single doses on consecutive days), 100 mg monthly or 150 mg monthly. At 1 year all monthly regimens were shown to be at least as good as the daily regimen in terms of changes in BMD at the spine and hip, and at the spine the 150 mg monthly regimen was superior to the daily regimen. This study has formed the basis for approval of once-monthly (150 mg) ibandronate.

In the DIVA (Dosing IntraVenous Administration) trial, intravenous ibandronate, 3 mg once every 3 months, or 2 mg once every 2 months, was non-inferior and statistically superior to oral ibandronate, 2.5 mg daily, in increasing lumbar spine BMD. Subsequent to these findings, the intravenous regimen of 3 mg every 3 months has been approved.

Tolerability. Ibandronate was well tolerated in clinical trials, with no significant excess of side effects in treated women when compared with placebo; women with a previous history of, or at risk from, upper gastrointestinal disease were not excluded from the studies. The dosing instructions require that the tablet is taken after an overnight fast (of at least 6 hours) and 1 hour before the first food or drink (other than water) of the day. The tablet should be swallowed whole with 180–240 ml of plain water while the patient is standing or sitting upright, and patients are instructed not to lie down for 1 hour after taking the tablet.

Dose and indication. Ibandronate is available as a single tablet, 150 mg, once monthly, or as an intravenous injection, 3 mg every 3 months, administered over 15–30 seconds. It is approved for the treatment of postmenopausal women to reduce the risk of vertebral fracture.

Zoledronate is a nitrogen-containing bisphosphonate recently approved for the treatment of osteoporosis in Europe and the USA.

Efficacy. The effects of annual infusions of zoledronate, 5 mg, were examined in the HORIZON study, a large randomized placebo-controlled trial in 7765 postmenopausal women with osteoporosis. After 3 years of treatment, morphometric vertebral fractures, hip fractures and all non-vertebral fractures were reduced by 70%, 41% and 25%, respectively, compared with placebo. Clinical vertebral fractures were reduced by 77% (Figure 7.4). Significant improvement in BMD at the spine and total hip was also demonstrated in the treatment group.

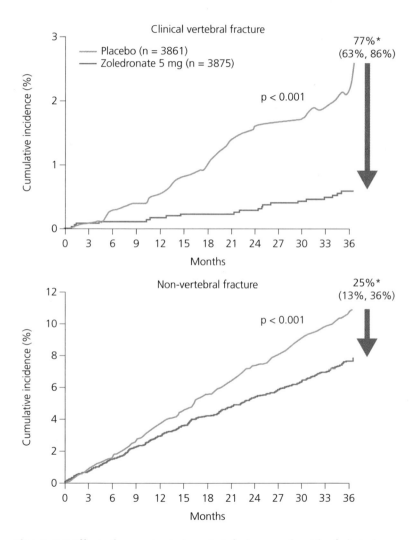

Figure 7.4 Effect of annual zoledronate infusions on the risk of clinical vertebral fractures and on non-vertebral fractures after 3 years of treatment in postmenopausal women with osteoporosis. Reproduced with permission from Black DM et al. 2007. Copyright © 2007 Massachusetts Medical Society. All rights reserved.

In another placebo-controlled trial, 2027 men and women who had recently sustained a hip fracture were randomized to receive annual infusions of zoledronate, 5 mg, or placebo. The rate of any new clinical fracture after a median follow-up period of 1.9 years was 8.6% in the treatment group and 13.9% in the placebo group. Treatment with zoledronate in this trial corresponded to an overall 35% reduction in fracture risk. Clinical vertebral fractures and all non-vertebral fractures were also significantly reduced (Figure 7.5) in zoledronate-treated patients and there was a significant increase in BMD in the femoral neck and total hip. Additionally, there was a 28% reduction in all-cause mortality in the patients treated with zoledronate compared with placebo.

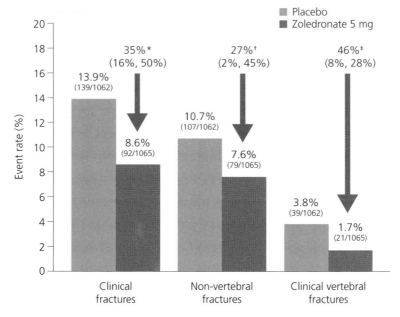

Figure 7.5 Effect on clinical fractures after 3 years of treatment with an annual infusion of zoledronate, 5 mg, in patients who had recently suffered a hip fracture. *p=0.0012; †p=0.0338; ‡p=0.0210, relative risk reduction vs placebo; NS, not significant. Values above bars are cumulative event rates based on Kaplan–Meier estimates at month 24. Reproduced with permission from Lyles et al. 2007. Copyright © 2007 Massachusetts Medical Society. All rights reserved.

Tolerability. With zoledronate infusions the most frequent adverse event is an acute phase reaction, in which a flu-like illness develops after the infusion, usually lasting 24–48 hours. This side effect is seen in around 30–40% of patients, but in most cases only occurs after the first infusion. In the HORIZON study, the risk of serious atrial fibrillation increased significantly in patients treated with zoledronate, although this was not seen in the other study referred to above, in which the patients had sustained a hip fracture and were older and frailer.

Dose and indication. Zoledronate, 5 mg, is given once yearly by intravenous infusion. The minimum duration of the infusion should be 15 minutes. The drug is approved for the treatment of osteoporosis in postmenopausal women at increased risk of fracture.

Etidronate sodium, the only drug in the first generation of bisphosphonates, is given cyclically – usually 2 weeks on and 3 months off – to reduce the possibility of inhibiting bone mineralization. Its use has been largely superseded by more potent bisphosphonates.

Efficacy. After 3–5 years of treatment, BMD in the lumbar vertebrae increases by 3–5%. In addition, in women with low BMD and prevalent fractures, etidronate may reduce the future incidence of spinal fractures.

Tolerability. In general, etidronate is well tolerated. The patient should be instructed to avoid food for 2 hours before and after taking the tablet. Cyclic etidronate/calcium therapy may be associated with gastrointestinal side effects, which are usually caused by the calcium supplements rather than etidronate.

Dose and indication. Cyclic etidronate is given 400 mg daily for 14 days, followed by calcium citrate, 500 mg daily for 76 days; the 90-day cycle is repeated as required. Etidronate sodium is licensed for both prevention and treatment of postmenopausal osteoporosis in the UK and some parts of Europe.

Possible adverse effects of bisphosphonate therapy

Osteonecrosis of the jaw (ONJ). An association between osteonecrosis of the jaw and high-dose bisphosphonate therapy has been documented in patients with cancer. However, it remains unclear whether the risk of ONJ is increased in non-cancer patients receiving lower doses of bisphosphonate for osteoporosis. The risk of developing ONJ is significantly increased in the presence of dental infection or oral trauma (e.g. tooth extraction), and most guidelines recommend that severe dental problems should be addressed before bisphosphonate therapy is started.

Femoral shaft fractures. A number of case reports have appeared over the past few years describing unusual fractures, particularly femoral shaft fractures, in patients with osteoporosis who had received treatment with a bisphosphonate. Prodromal pain is a characteristic feature of these fractures, which often fail to heal normally. A causal association with bisphosphonate therapy has not been definitely established but cannot be excluded.

Selective estrogen-receptor modulators

The selective estrogen-receptor modulators interact with the estrogen receptor, but in a different way from estrogen, resulting in mixed agonist and antagonist effects in different tissues.

Raloxifene. In healthy perimenopausal women, raloxifene has been shown to prevent menopausal bone loss, with small gains in bone mass at the spine and hip and for the whole body.

Efficacy. The results of a randomized controlled trial in 7705 postmenopausal women with osteoporosis (the Multiple Outcomes of Raloxifene or MORE study) have shown that raloxifene increases BMD in the spine and hip. After 3 years of treatment with raloxifene, 60 mg daily, the risk of vertebral fracture was reduced by 30% overall; the reduction was 30% in women with a vertebral fracture at baseline, and 50% in those without (Figure 7.6). Clinical vertebral fractures were reduced within 1 year of starting treatment, and a reduction in vertebral fractures was also shown in a subset of postmenopausal women with osteopenia rather than osteoporosis. However, no significant reduction in non-vertebral fractures was demonstrated in this study.

Tolerability. Unlike HRT, raloxifene does not stimulate the endometrium and therefore is not associated with increased frequency of vaginal bleeding or increased risk of endometrial cancer.

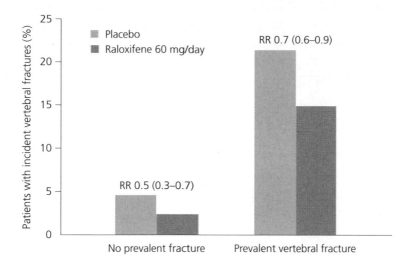

Figure 7.6 Effect of raloxifene on vertebral fracture: the Multiple Outcomes of Raloxifene (MORE) study. RR, relative risk. Data from Ettinger et al. 1999.

A significant reduction in the risk of invasive breast cancer has been demonstrated in women taking raloxifene for up to 4 years, for all breast cancers (RR 0.28; 95% CI 0.17–0.46) and for estrogen-receptor-positive breast cancers (RR 0.16; 95% CI 0.09–0.30).

Raloxifene has favorable effects on serum lipids similar to those seen with estrogen, but its effects on cardiovascular disease morbidity and mortality are not yet known, although a large study is under way to investigate this. Similarly, the effects of raloxifene on cognitive function remain to be defined.

Raloxifene does not alleviate, and may exacerbate, vasomotor menopausal symptoms and thus is not suitable for perimenopausal women with active symptoms. Side effects are generally mild and include hot flashes, leg edema and leg cramps. There is an approximately three-fold increase in the relative risk of venous thromboembolism, similar to that seen with HRT and with tamoxifen. A recent study also demonstrated a small increase in the risk of stroke in raloxifene-treated women.

Dose and indication. Raloxifene is licensed for the prevention and treatment of postmenopausal osteoporosis when administered orally as a single daily dose of 60 mg. It is a useful treatment option in postmenopausal women with vertebral osteoporosis and in those who are intolerant of other therapies. In view of the lack of evidence for efficacy against hip fracture, however, it is less suitable for elderly women in whom the risk of hip fracture is high.

Hormone replacement therapy

The role of estrogen deficiency in the pathogenesis of osteoporosis is well documented, and estrogen replacement has, until recently, been widely used in the prevention of osteoporotic fractures. In conventional doses, estrogen acts as an antiresorptive agent, although high doses have been shown to have anabolic skeletal effects.

Hormone replacement preparations. The term HRT is used to describe two types of preparation:
- estrogen-only (unopposed) therapy
- combined estrogen and progestogen (opposed or combined) therapy.

Since unopposed-estrogen therapy confers an increased risk of endometrial hyperplasia and cancer, progestogens are usually given for a minimum of 10–14 days of each monthly cycle in women with an intact uterus. Estrogens may be given continuously or intermittently (for 21 out of 28 days) in unopposed or combined preparations. Oral, transdermal and subcutaneously implanted preparations have all been shown to be effective in the prevention of bone loss. However, absorption from vaginal preparations does not give adequate protection against bone loss.

Efficacy. HRT, whether unopposed or combined, prevents menopausal bone loss in the spine, femur and radius. Until recently, most of the evidence for fracture reduction was derived from observational studies; however, significant reduction in clinical vertebral and non-vertebral fractures was reported from the Women's Health Initiative study, a large, randomized controlled trial in healthy postmenopausal women.

Tolerability. The most troublesome short-term side effect of HRT is vaginal bleeding, which is a major cause of poor compliance, particularly in more elderly women. Other short-term side effects include breast tenderness, nausea, dyspepsia, bloating, headache and mood changes.

Recent evidence indicates that HRT is not protective against coronary heart disease, as was previously believed; furthermore, HRT has been shown to increase the risk of stroke, as well as the known increase in risk of breast cancer and venous thromboembolic disease.

The general consensus is that, despite protection against osteoporosis (and also colon cancer), the risk–benefit profile is unfavorable for the majority of postmenopausal women (Table 7.1) and HRT should be regarded as a second-line option for the treatment of osteoporosis.

TABLE 7.1

Risk–benefit balance for healthy postmenopausal women taking hormone replacement therapy for 5 years

Total excess of adverse effects (breast cancer, stroke, pulmonary embolism)

- Women aged 50–59 years   1 in 170 users
- Women aged 60–69 years   1 in 80 users

Total excess of benefits (colorectal cancer, hip fracture)

- Women aged 50–59 years   1 in 600 users
- Women aged 60–69 years   1 in 180 users

Note that the absolute risk of adverse effects increases with age, as a result of an increase in the background incidence of those conditions. Likewise, the probability of benefit increases with age. Nevertheless, in healthy postmenopausal women the risks of long-term treatment generally outweigh the benefits. Data from Beral V et al. Copyright © 2002, with permission from Elsevier.

Other antiresorptive agents

Calcitonin is a naturally occurring 22-amino-acid polypeptide produced by parafollicular cells in the thyroid. It increases calcium excretion in the kidney and inhibits bone resorption by acting directly at the receptor located on the osteoclast, thereby leading to a secondary increase in BMD.

As interspecies differences are quite minimal and salmon calcitonin (sCT) is one of the most potent and readily available peptides, it has been used in almost all clinical trials of calcitonin in osteoporosis. Parenteral and intranasal preparations of sCT are available in the USA and some other parts of the world, and are approved for the prevention and treatment of postmenopausal osteoporosis. Treatment with continuous parenteral sCT results in transient increases in lumbar BMD averaging 2–4% over 2 years, whereas femoral neck and hip BMD show little or no change. Intranasal sCT, 200 IU/day, which is now in use in some European countries and the USA, possesses some analgesic properties. In addition, a recent study has shown a reduction in vertebral fractures in women with postmenopausal osteoporosis treated with intranasal sCT, 200 IU/day; this reduction was associated with very small changes in BMD, similar to those seen in the control group. No significant decrease was seen in women treated with 100 or 400 IU/day.

Although parenteral sCT has been associated with flashing (known as 'flushing' in the UK) and nausea, intranasal sCT has almost no side effects. However, the potential of either of these sCTs to increase BMD is less than that of either HRT or bisphosphonates. In addition, data on antifracture efficacy are inconsistent.

Calcium with or without vitamin D. Calcium supplementation has antiresorptive effects because it suppresses endogenous production of parathyroid hormone (PTH), thereby reducing an important stimulus to bone remodeling. Both dietary calcium intake and calcium supplementation to more than 1000 mg/day are effective in reducing PTH concentrations and thereby reducing bone loss in older postmenopausal women.

Beneficial effects of calcium supplementation on BMD have been demonstrated in children and adults, particularly at appendicular

Key points – antiresorptive therapy

- The bisphosphonates alendronate, risedronate and zoledronate reduce fracture at vertebral and non-vertebral sites, including the hip, in postmenopausal women with osteoporosis.
- Ibandronate, another bisphosphonate, is also approved for the treatment of postmenopausal osteoporosis although reduction in hip fractures has not been demonstrated.
- Raloxifene, a selective estrogen-receptor modulator, reduces vertebral fracture risk in postmenopausal women with osteoporosis.
- HRT has been shown to reduce clinical vertebral and non-vertebral fractures, including hip fractures, in healthy postmenopausal women, but the adverse effects of long-term treatment restrict its use for osteoporosis.
- The evidence base for the antifracture efficacy of calcitonin and calcitriol is less secure.
- Calcium and vitamin D supplementation reduces non-vertebral fractures, including hip fractures, in very elderly individuals living in residential accommodation but not in the free-living elderly population.
- Calcium and vitamin D supplements should be given as an adjunct to other pharmacological interventions unless there is clear evidence that calcium intake and vitamin D status are adequate.

skeletal sites; in the spine, these effects are less evident and may be transient. Furthermore, the beneficial skeletal effects of calcium are reduced in perimenopausal women, in whom the principal mechanism for bone loss is estrogen deficiency. There is no robust evidence from randomized controlled trials that calcium supplementation reduces fracture risk.

Evidence from a study of nursing-home residents strongly suggests that calcium supplementation plus vitamin D, 800 IU/day, can reduce the number of hip fractures and prevent age-related bone loss.

However, recent studies in free-living elderly populations have failed to demonstrate efficacy of vitamin D ± calcium supplements in either the primary or secondary prevention of fractures.

A study among postmenopausal women in New Zealand has suggested that the active form of vitamin D, 1,25-dihydroxyvitamin D3, given with calcium, reduces the incidence of vertebral fractures, though the design of this study was suboptimal and other studies of this vitamin D metabolite have failed to demonstrate efficacy against fractures.

Overall, current evidence does not support the use of calcium and vitamin D supplementation as a definitive treatment for osteoporosis, except in the frail elderly population living in residential care. However, it should be considered as an adjunct to other therapies with proven antifracture efficacy, because all patients assessed in the randomized controlled trials of these agents were calcium and vitamin D replete. Furthermore, there is evidence that vitamin D supplementation has beneficial effects on muscle strength and reduces the likelihood of falling. Thus, daily supplementation with calcium (around 1 g) and vitamin D (400–800 IU) should be given to all individuals treated with pharmacotherapy for osteoporosis, unless there is clear evidence that calcium intake and vitamin D status are adequate.

Key references

Beral V, Banks E, Reeves G. Evidence from randomised trials on the long-term effects of hormone replacement therapy. *Lancet* 2002;360:942–44.

Black DM, Cummings SR, Karpf DB et al. Randomised trial of the effect of alendronate on risk of fracture in women with existing vertebral fractures. Fracture Intervention Trial Research Group. *Lancet* 1996;348: 1535–41.

Black DM, Delmas PD, Eastell R et al. Once-yearly zoledronic acid for treatment of postmenopausal osteoporosis. *New Engl J Med* 2007;356:1809–22.

Chapuy MC, Arlot ME, DuBoeuf F et al. Vitamin D3 and calcium to prevent hip fractures in elderly women. *N Engl J Med* 1992;327: 1637–42.

Chesnut CH 3rd, Skag A, Christiansen C et al. Effects of oral ibandronate administered daily or intermittently on fracture risk in postmenopausal osteoporosis. *J Bone Miner Res* 2004;19:1241–9.

Ettinger B, Black DM, Mitlak BH et al. Reduction of vertebral risk in postmenopausal women with osteoporosis treated with raloxifene: results from a 3-year randomized clinical trial. Multiple Outcomes of Raloxifene Evaluation (MORE) Investigators. *JAMA* 1999;282: 637–45.

Grant AM, Avenell A, Campbell MK et al. Oral vitamin D3 and calcium for secondary prevention of low-trauma fractures in elderly people (Randomised Evaluation of Calcium Or vitamin D, RECORD): a randomised placebo-controlled trial. *Lancet* 2005;365:1621–8.

Harris ST, Watts NB, Genant HK et al. Effects of risedronate treatment on vertebral and nonvertebral fractures in women with postmenopausal osteoporosis: a randomized controlled trial. Vertebral Efficacy with Risedronate Therapy (VERT) Study Group. *JAMA* 1999;282:1344–52.

Khan AA, Sandor GK, Dore E et al. Canadian consensus practice guidelines for bisphosphonate associated osteonecrosis of the jaw. *J Rheumatol* 2008;35:1391–7.

Lyles KW, Colon-Emeric CS, Magaziner JS et al. Zoledronic acid and clinical fractures and mortality after hip fracture. *N Engl J Med* 2007;357:1799–809.

McClung MR, Geusens P, Miller PD et al. Effect of risedronate on the risk of hip fracture in elderly women. Hip Intervention Program Study Group. *N Engl J Med* 2001;344:333–40.

Miller PD, McClung MR, Macovei L et al. Monthly oral ibandronate therapy in postmenopausal osteoporosis: 1-year results from the MOBILE study. *J Bone Miner Res* 2005;20:1315–22.

Poole KE, Compston JE. Osteoporosis and its management. *BMJ* 2006;333:1251–6.

Porthouse J, Cockayne S, King C et al. Randomised controlled trial of calcium supplementation with cholecalciferol (vitamin D3) for prevention of fractures in primary care. *BMJ* 2005;330:1003.

Reginster J-Y, Minne HW, Sorensen OH et al. Randomized trial of the effects of risedronate on vertebral fractures in women with established postmenopausal osteoporosis. Vertebral Efficacy with Risedronate Therapy (VERT) Study Group. *Osteoporos Int* 2000;11: 83–91.

Strontium ranelate and parathyroid hormone peptides

Other drugs used for osteoporosis act differently from antiresorptives, by stimulating bone turnover and bone formation and/or altering bone composition.

Strontium ranelate

Strontium ranelate acts differently from other bone-protective interventions, strengthening bone by a mechanism that is believed to involve changes in the bone matrix/mineral composite and maintaining bone formation in association with reduced resorption. Strontium is a bone-seeking element that is taken up by bone, mainly by adsorption to the surface of hydroxyapatite crystals. There is limited exchange of strontium with the calcium in hydroxyapatite, with a maximum replacement by strontium when given in high doses of one in every ten calcium atoms. Strontium ranelate contains two atoms of stable strontium and an organic acid anion, ranelate.

Efficacy. Long-term results of two large Phase III studies investigating the effects of strontium ranelate have recently been reported: SOTI (Spinal Osteoporosis Therapeutic Intervention) and TROPOS (TReatment Of Peripheral OSteoporosis).

In SOTI, the effects on vertebral fracture reduction were investigated in 1649 postmenopausal women with established osteoporosis. Women treated with strontium ranelate showed a 41% reduction in relative risk (RR) over 3 years. The proportion of treated women with a new vertebral fracture over 3 years was 20.9%, compared with 32.8% of women who received placebo. The beneficial effect on vertebral fracture was seen after only 1 year of treatment: 6.4% of treated women had a vertebral fracture compared with 12.2% of women who received placebo. Efficacy was sustained over 4 years of treatment with a 33% reduction in vertebral fractures (Figure 8.1). There was also significantly less height loss in women treated with strontium ranelate.

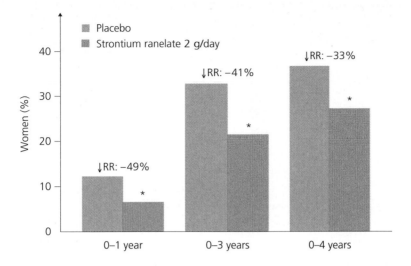

Figure 8.1 Long-term effect of strontium ranelate on the risk of vertebral fracture (SOTI results). Significant reductions were seen in postmenopausal women treated with strontium ranelate, 2 g/day, after 1, 3 and 4 years of treatment (49%, 41% and 33% reductions in risk, respectively). *Statistically significant difference from placebo; $p < 0.001$. RR, relative risk. Data from Meunier et al. 2004 and 2009.

In TROPOS, fracture reduction was investigated in 5091 postmenopausal women with osteoporosis. Uniquely, sustained efficacy of strontium ranelate against both vertebral and non-vertebral fractures was demonstrated over 5 years, with a significant (15%) reduction in all non-vertebral fractures; the results for women at high risk of hip fracture showed a significant (43%) reduction in hip fracture after 5 years. The risk of vertebral fracture was reduced by 24% compared with placebo over this period (Figure 8.2).

Furthermore, analysis in women aged 80 years or older has shown significant antifracture efficacy at both vertebral and non-vertebral sites, with maintenance of efficacy over 5 years.

Lumbar spine BMD increased significantly in women treated with strontium ranelate in both SOTI and TROPOS; after correction for the effect of bone strontium on the measurement, the mean increase relative to placebo was approximately 8% after 3 years of treatment. There

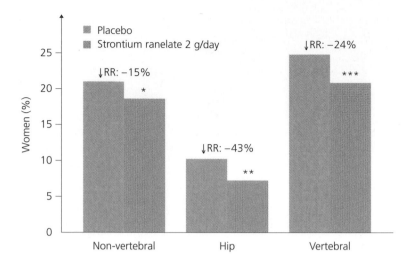

Figure 8.2 Effect of strontium ranelate on the risk of non-vertebral fracture, hip fracture and vertebral fracture after 5 years (TROPOS results). Fracture risk was significantly reduced by 15%, 43% and 24%, respectively. *Statistically significant difference from placebo: *p = 0.032; **p = 0.036; ***p < 0.001. RR, relative risk. Data from Reginster et al. 2008.

were also significant increases in femoral neck BMD relative to placebo.

Tolerability. In trials, the overall incidence for adverse events with strontium ranelate did not differ from placebo, and adverse events were usually mild and transient.

Dose and indication. Strontium ranelate is taken orally in a daily 2 g dose. It has been approved in Europe for the prevention of vertebral and hip fractures in postmenopausal women with osteoporosis.

Parathyroid hormone peptides

Teriparatide. Parathyroid hormone (PTH) (1-34, teriparatide) administered intermittently has now been shown to have dramatic effects on the skeleton, with some changes evident within the first 4 weeks of treatment. During the past decade, tremendous progress has also been made in understanding and clarifying its mode of action.

As long as 50 years ago, scientists observed that native PTH could stimulate bone formation in vitro and in experimental animals when administered intermittently. It had also been shown to increase bone density, strength and connectivity in small trials in both humans and animals.

Efficacy. In a randomized controlled trial of 1637 women with established osteoporosis, the effects of teriparatide, 20 µg or 40 µg administered daily by subcutaneous injection, were examined over a mean treatment period of 18 months. There were significant increases in BMD in the spine and proximal femur. The study results also showed significant reductions of 65–70% in vertebral fractures and of 53–54% in non-vertebral fractures (Figure 8.3). The risk of two or more new vertebral fractures was reduced by 77% in the 20 µg group and 86% in the 40 µg group. The risk of at least one moderate or severe vertebral fracture was reduced by 90% and 78% in the 20 µg and 40 µg groups,

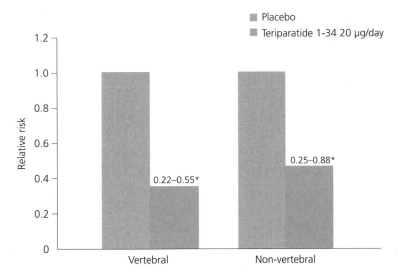

Figure 8.3 Effect of recombinant human parathyroid hormone peptide 1-34 (teriparatide) on the risk for vertebral and non-vertebral fractures in postmenopausal women with established osteoporosis. Women received teriparatide, 20 µg daily by subcutaneous injection, or placebo for a median period of 18 months. *95% confidence interval. Data from Neer et al. 2001.

respectively. There was also a significant decrease in new or worsening back pain in the two treatment groups: 23% placebo versus 17% (20 μg) and 16% (40 μg). The beneficial effect of teriparatide on vertebral fractures was largely independent of age, baseline BMD and the status of prevalent vertebral fractures. In fact, no cases of osteosarcoma have been reported in humans even after careful postmarketing surveillance. In addition, no association between primary hyperparathyroidism and the development of osteosarcoma has been found in several very large series.

Tolerability. Teriparatide, when used in the approved dose of 20 μg daily, was not associated with severe adverse effects in the Phase III clinical trial described above; only dizziness and nausea were slightly more common in the treatment group than in the placebo group.

Transient mild hypercalcemia occurs within 4–6 hours of the injection, but routine monitoring of serum calcium is not required.

An increased incidence of osteosarcoma was observed in preclinical toxicology experiments in rats, but is not thought to be relevant to the short-term use of lower doses (20 μg/day for 18 months) in postmenopausal women.

Dose and indication. The recommended dose for teriparatide is 20 μg daily, administered subcutaneously into the thigh or abdomen from a prefilled pen. In Europe, the treatment period is usually limited to a maximum of 18 months, and in the USA to 12–18 months.

Teriparatide is more expensive than other treatments and is most widely used in women with severe osteoporosis who are intolerant of or unresponsive to other interventions. Also, it should be noted that after discontinuation of PTH bone density starts to decline. Hence, treatment with PTH followed by an antiresorptive seems the most appropriate regimen for long-term intervention.

PTH 1-84 has been shown to reduce vertebral fractures, and has been approved in Europe for the treatment of postmenopausal osteoporosis in women at high risk of fractures. The recommended dose is 100 μg/day by subcutaneous injection into the abdomen.

Key points – strontium ranelate and parathyroid hormone peptides

- Strontium ranelate's mechanism of action is believed to involve changes in the bone matrix/mineral composite, promoting bone strength and maintaining bone formation.
- In postmenopausal women with osteoporosis, strontium ranelate has demonstrated efficacy, sustained over 5 years, in the reduction of vertebral and non-vertebral fractures, and hip fractures in high-risk women.
- Parathyroid hormone (PTH) has anabolic effects on bone when administered intermittently.
- Teriparatide (recombinant human PTH peptide 1-34), administered by daily subcutaneous injection, produces large increases in bone mineral density (BMD), and reduces vertebral and non-vertebral fractures in postmenopausal women with osteoporosis.

Key references

Black DM, Bilezikian JP, Ensrud KE et al. One year of alendronate after one year of parathyroid hormone (1-84) for osteoporosis. *N Engl J Med* 2005;353:555–65.

Marie PJ, Ammann P, Boivin G, Rey C. Mechanisms of action and therapeutic potential of strontium in bone. *Calcif Tissue Int* 2001;69:121–9.

Meunier PJ, Roux C, Ortolani S et al. Effects of long-term strontium ranelate treatment on vertebral fracture risk in postmenopausal women with osteoporosis. *Osteoporos Int* 2009;Jan 20 [Epub ahead of print].

Meunier PJ, Roux C, Seeman E et al. The effects of strontium ranelate on the risk of vertebral fracture in women with postmenopausal osteoporosis. *N Engl J Med* 2004; 350:459–68.

Meunier PJ, Slosman DO, Delmas PD et al. Strontium ranelate: dose-dependent effects in established postmenopausal vertebral osteoporosis – a 2-year randomized placebo controlled trial. *J Clin Endocr Metab* 2002;87:2060–6.

Neer RM, Arnaud CD, Zanchetta JR et al. Effect of parathyroid hormone (1-34) on fractures and bone mineral density in postmenopausal women with osteoporosis. *N Engl J Med* 2001;344:1434–41.

Reginster J-Y, Felsenberg D, Boonen S et al. Effects of long-term strontium ranelate treatment on the risk of nonvertebral and vertebral fractures in postmenopausal osteoporosis. *Arthritis Rheum* 2008;58:1687–95.

Seeman E, Vellas B, Benhamou C et al. Strontium ranelate reduces the risk of vertebral and nonvertebral fractures in women eighty years of age and older. *J Bone Miner Res* 2006;21:1113–20.

Zanchetta JR, Bogado CE, Ferretti JL et al. Effects of teriparatide [recombinant human parathyroid hormone (1-34)] on cortical bone in postmenopausal women with osteoporosis. *J Bone Miner Res* 2003;18:539–43.

Glucocorticoid-induced osteoporosis

Glucocorticoid-induced osteoporosis is one of the most common forms of the disorder, and has a multifactorial etiology (see Figure 2.6, page 22). Studies using the General Practice Research Database in the UK have provided important new information about this condition.

- Even small daily doses of oral prednisolone (< 7.5 mg) are associated with increased fracture risk (Figure 9.1).
- After oral glucocorticoid therapy is initiated, fracture risk increases rapidly (in the first 3–6 months) (Figure 9.2). This fast response to glucocorticoid therapy emphasizes the importance of early prevention of osteoporosis in high-risk patients.
- After glucocorticoid therapy is stopped, fracture risk decreases towards baseline values.

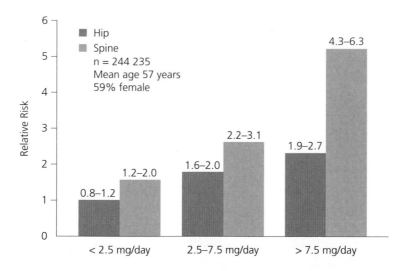

Figure 9.1 Use of oral glucocorticoids and relative risk of hip and spine fracture. Note that even at daily doses of less than 7.5 mg prednisolone, fracture risk is increased. 95% confidence intervals are given above each column. Data from van Staa et al. 2000.

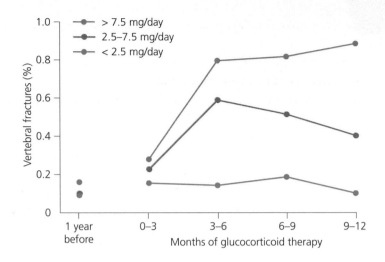

Figure 9.2 Time course of vertebral fractures during oral glucocorticoid therapy. Note the rapid rise in fracture incidence during the first 3–6 months in the high- and intermediate-dose groups. Data from van Staa et al. 2000.

Treatment options concentrate on preventing further bone loss and reducing or eliminating glucocorticoid therapy to the level necessary to suppress the underlying disease process.

Several randomized placebo-controlled trials have demonstrated the efficacy of first- and second-generation bisphosphonates in the prevention of bone loss in men and women receiving glucocorticoids. Cyclic etidronate, 400 mg daily for 2 weeks every 3 months, alendronate, 10 mg daily, and risedronate, 5 mg daily, can maintain spine and hip bone mass despite persistent glucocorticoid therapy. In addition, there is evidence that these therapies reduce the risk of new vertebral fractures in glucocorticoid-treated postmenopausal women. Thus, bisphosphonates are the first-line option for the prevention and treatment of glucocorticoid-induced osteoporosis. Teriparatide has also been shown to prevent bone loss in glucocorticoid-treated men and women and is approved for this indication in Europe and the USA.

As in postmenopausal osteoporosis, administration of adequate calcium and vitamin D is important as an adjunct to bisphosphonate therapy.

Hypogonadism, where present, should be corrected.

Finally, since rapid bone loss is very common when glucocorticoids and immunosuppressants are administered after organ transplantation, bisphosphonates may, in this population, be the treatment of choice to prevent osteoporotic fractures.

Evidence-based guidelines in the UK recommend that men and women over the age of 65 years or with a previous history of fragility fracture should be offered bone protective therapy when glucocorticoid therapy is initiated, with no need for bone densitometry beforehand.

In other glucocorticoid-treated patients, intervention should be advised if a fragility fracture occurs or if the bone mineral density (BMD) T-score is below –1.5. However, age should be taken into consideration when making treatment decisions, since the absolute risk of fracture is low in the majority of young individuals; furthermore, bisphosphonates cross the placenta and should therefore be used with caution in premenopausal women.

Osteoporosis in men

Osteoporotic fractures in men are becoming an increasing problem as a result of the aging of the population and are associated with a higher mortality than in women. Secondary causes of osteoporosis are common, particularly glucocorticoid therapy, alcohol abuse and hypogonadism. Bone loss in older men is closely related to estrogen status; in addition, vitamin D insufficiency and secondary hyperparathyroidism are likely to contribute.

As in postmenopausal women, there is a strong relationship between BMD and fracture risk in men. Whether sex-specific reference ranges should be used to define the T-score remains an issue for debate, and this is reflected in guidelines from different parts of the world.

Treatment options. A randomized controlled trial has shown that alendronate, 10 mg daily, results in significant increases in BMD in the spine and proximal femur of men with osteoporosis. Vertebral fractures were also reduced after the 2-year treatment period. In addition, data from a 2-year trial of risedronate, 35 mg weekly, showed significant improvements in lumbar spine BMD at 6, 12 and 24 months. Both of these regimens are now licensed in Europe and the USA for the treatment of osteoporosis in men. Teriparatide has also been shown to have beneficial effects on BMD in men with osteoporosis and is now approved for this indication in Europe and the USA.

As with other forms of osteoporosis, calcium and vitamin D supplementation should be recommended as adjunctive therapy unless there is evidence of adequate calcium intake and normal vitamin D status.

Key points – other forms of osteoporosis

- Oral glucocorticoid therapy is an important cause of osteoporosis; fracture risk increases at all doses of oral prednisolone and rises rapidly during the first 3–6 months of therapy.
- Alendronate, risedronate and teriparatide are approved for the treatment of glucocorticoid-induced osteoporosis.
- Primary prevention should be offered to all high-risk patients taking oral glucocorticoids for 3 months or more (e.g. men and women over 65 years and those with a previous fragility fracture).
- Osteoporosis in men is an increasing problem.
- Alendronate, risedronate and teriparatide are approved for the treatment of men with osteoporosis.

Key references

Adachi JD, Bensen WG, Brown J et al. Intermittent etidronate therapy to prevent corticosteroid-induced osteoporosis. N Engl J Med 1997; 337:382–7.

Cohen S, Levy RM, Keller M et al. Risedronate therapy prevents corticosteroid-induced bone loss: a twelve-month, multicenter, randomized, double-blind, placebo-controlled, parallel-group study. Arthritis Rheum 1999;42:2309–18.

Kanis JA, Johansson H, Oden A et al. A meta-analysis of prior corticosteroid use and fracture risk. *J Bone Miner Res* 2004;19:893–9.

Khosla S, Amin S, Orwoll E. Osteoporosis in men. *Endocr Rev* 2008;29:441–64.

Orwoll E, Ettinger M, Weiss S et al. Alendronate for the treatment of osteoporosis in men. *N Engl J Med* 2000;343:604–10.

Reid DM, Hughes RA, Laan RF et al. Efficacy and safety of daily risedronate in the treatment of corticosteroid-induced osteoporosis in men and women: a randomized trial. European Corticosteroid-Induced Osteoporosis Treatment Study. *J Bone Miner Res* 2000;15:1006–13.

Saag KG, Emkey R, Schnitzer TJ et al. Alendronate for the prevention and treatment of glucocorticoid-induced osteoporosis. Gluocorticoid-Induced Osteoporosis Intervention Study Group. *N Engl J Med* 1998; 339:292–9.

Saag KG, Shane E, Boonen S et al. Teriparatide or alendronate in glucocorticoid-induced osteoporosis. *New Engl J Med* 2007;357:2028–39.

van Staa TP, Leufkens HG, Abenhaim L et al. Use of oral corticosteroids and risk of fractures. *J Bone Miner Res* 2000;15:993–1000.

van Staa TP, Leufkens HGM, Cooper C. The epidemiology of corticosteroid-induced osteoporosis: a meta-analysis. *Osteoporos Int* 2002;13:777–87.

10 Future trends

The number of osteoporotic fractures is expected to increase dramatically over the next 50 years. In particular, it is forecast that by the year 2050 the number of hip fractures will double in North American women, and will almost quadruple among Latin American and Asian women. This increase is partly due to improvements in healthcare that have increased life expectancy. In addition, technological advances will almost certainly increase the number of people identified as being at risk.

Despite the increasing prevalence of this disease, the future bodes well for earlier diagnosis and more promising treatment.

Diagnosis

The use of dual-energy X-ray absorptiometry as a diagnostic technique has risen and is likely to continue to do so. Meanwhile, less costly techniques to measure bone mass, such as ultrasound of the heel and radiogrammetry, have recently become available and are likely to be used for screening. In the future, techniques to enable more rapid measurement (e.g. scanning of a single finger) may provide almost instantaneous assessment of fracture risk. However, probably the biggest advance in the field will come from perfecting non-invasive measures of bone quality. These will include peripheral quantitative computed tomography (QCT) of the radius and tibia, QCT of the spine and femur, and magnetic resonance imaging of the radius and calcaneus. An integrated measure of both quality and quantity is likely to improve our ability to assess fracture risk accurately.

Biochemical markers of bone turnover, such as urinary and serum collagen crosslinks, skeletal alkaline phosphatase and procollagen peptides, could emerge as important predictors of bone loss, as well as being used to ascertain the magnitude of response to antiresorptive therapy.

New methods of carrying out these assays will make it easy to perform capillary analysis of fracture risk. Soon, multichannel colorimetric analyses of serum samples will provide risk assessments for both heart disease (via cholesterol) and osteoporosis at very low cost. In coming years, family physicians may be able to provide perimenopausal patients with a relatively accurate prediction of fracture risk based on a single measurement of bone mass and one or two biochemical indices of bone turnover.

However, this prediction is based on the likelihood that new biochemical markers of turnover will become commercially available. Tartrate-resistant acid phosphatase 5b, a sensitive serum marker of bone resorption, is one such test that may be useful for early diagnosis of rapid bone loss, as well as being a potential indicator of metastatic bone disease.

Genetic analysis. Bone density is a polygenic trait, and genetic screening for osteoporotic risk is beginning to emerge as a future tool. To date, polymorphisms in several candidate genes have been associated with bone mass, although, in general, the strength of the association has been relatively weak. This weak association suggests that multiple genes contribute to the BMD phenotype. Recent research has identified a polymorphism in the *BMP-2* gene as having a strong association with fracture in Icelandic women. As more genes are identified, screening for several genes in capillary blood, hair or saliva may become commonplace.

Several of the genes that influence the development of osteoporosis are thought to be modified by environmental factors. Early identification of a genetic predisposition to the disease would enable prophylactic intervention (e.g. calcium supplementation, exercise, HRT) to optimize the peak bone mass attained and thereby help to prevent osteoporosis.

As well as influencing acquisition of peak bone mass, genes may also be important in defining the rate of bone loss during and immediately after menopause. Genetic profiling may therefore prove useful in the future in helping to define those at greatest risk of fracture.

Selection of patients for treatment

Evidence suggests that interventions used to prevent osteoporotic fractures have a relatively rapid rate of onset and offset of treatment effect. Several interventions have been shown to produce significant reductions in fracture rate after only 1 year of treatment, but beneficial effects on BMD, and probably also fracture, begin to wear off after treatment withdrawal. These observations, together with increasing recognition that worthwhile reductions in fracture rate can be achieved even in those with advanced bone loss and/or established osteoporosis, have resulted in a shift from preventive strategies in women with normal or only slightly reduced BMD to treatments that target high-risk individuals. These strategies have important cost implications because of the greater number of fractures prevented in high-risk than in low-risk populations, and the shorter duration of therapy required. Since the number of women at high risk increases with age, a case may be made for screening (using bone densitometry and risk factors) all women aged 65 years or over. Conversely, in women aged 80 years or more, in whom low BMD is almost always present and risk factors for falling are common, there is a strong argument for universal treatment, provided that the intervention is safe and relatively inexpensive.

New drug treatments

Several new approaches to osteoporosis therapy are emerging.

Selective estrogen-receptor modulators (SERMs). Several new SERMs are being developed, each with a distinct tissue-selective activity. However, most of these new agents have demonstrated non-skeletal side effects, such as uterine prolapse or hypertrophy, which may limit their clinical utility in the future. The ideal SERM, which would provide positive effects on bone, cardiovascular system and brain while suppressing tissue growth in the breast and uterus, has not yet reached clinical testing. The long-term effects of these drugs are unknown, and multisystem evaluations will be required for years to come. Currently, only raloxifene and tamoxifen are available.

Anabolic agents. Although there was a flurry of activity with growth hormone and insulin-like growth factor I in the mid-1990s, there is now sufficient evidence to suggest that these recombinant peptides will not be widely used, or even approved by regulatory agencies.

On the other hand, parathyroid hormone (PTH) (1-34 and 1-84) has an exciting future. PTH 1-84, 100 µg/day, which has been shown to reduce spine fractures by 60%, has now been approved in Europe for the treatment of postmenopausal osteoporosis. In addition, PTH may also be effective in glucocorticoid-induced osteoporosis, as it has been shown that daily injections of PTH increase bone mass in women taking glucocorticoids and HRT by up to 15% over 2 years. Larger studies in glucocorticoid-induced osteoporosis are indicated.

RANK ligand inhibitors. AMG 162 is a synthetic antibody to RANK ligand; it inhibits bone resorption and is administered twice yearly. Studies have shown significant increases in BMD with this well-tolerated agent. In one recent head-to-head trial the increase in BMD of the spine was greater with AMG 162 than with alendronate. Phase III trials are under way.

Parathyroid hormone rp (PTHrp) is a PTH-like product that occupies the same receptor as PTH and, when given intermittently, can stimulate bone formation. As with native PTH, PTHrp 1-36, administered daily as a subcutaneous injection, caused a 5% increase in spine BMD after only 3 months of treatment. Moreover, there were no changes in markers of bone resorption in this trial. Paradoxically, PTHrp is secreted by tumors and is one cause of severe malignant hypercalcemia. Further studies are needed to distinguish PTH from PTHrp and to determine where it might fit in the clinical armamentarium of therapies for osteoporosis.

Less certain is the role of combination therapy using both anabolic and antiresorptive agents. Recently published results suggest that concurrent use of PTH and alendronate is no better than PTH alone. In one study, PTH followed by alendronate was reported to increase bone mass in the spine by 14% over 2 years. Whether other antiresorptive agents, particularly drugs such as AMG 162, behave like alendronate in combination with PTH remains to be seen, and the issue of adding PTH to the therapeutic regimen of a patient already taking a bisphosphonate remains to be clarified.

Patient management

The dramatic rise in the prevalence of osteoporosis will undoubtedly overwhelm current healthcare resources. Furthermore, rapid advances in technology and treatment will challenge primary care providers to be at the forefront of both diagnosis and treatment. As the number of specialists treating osteoporosis begins to level off, or even decline, it will become vital for primary care physicians to form collaborations that will provide safe yet cost-effective delivery of healthcare services to a growing number of patients. It will become increasingly important for specialists in metabolic bone diseases to disseminate new information to their primary care colleagues and to facilitate a positive and evolving partnership to ensure that comprehensive care continues for patients with osteoporosis.

Key points – future trends

- The prevalence of osteoporosis is increasing, particularly in developing countries.
- New methods for imaging bone architecture are likely to improve diagnostic capabilities and risk assessments.
- Anabolic drugs offer great potential for use either alone or in sequence with bisphosphonates.

Key references

Black DM, Greenspan SL, Ensrud KE et al. The effects of parathyroid hormone and alendronate alone or in combination in postmenopausal osteoporosis. N Engl J Med 2003; 349:1207–15.

Bouxsein ML. Bone quality: where do we go from here? Osteoporos Int 2003;14(suppl 5):118–27.

Cummings SR, Melton LJ. Epidemiology and outcomes of osteoporotic fractures. *Lancet* 2002;359:1761–7.

Finkelstein JS, Hayes A, Hunzelman JL et al. The effects of parathyroid hormone, alendronate, or both in men with osteoporosis. *N Engl J Med* 2003;349:1216–26.

Klein RF, Allard J, Avnur Z et al. Regulation of bone mass in mice by the lipoxygenase gene Alox15. *Science* 2004;303:229–32.

Lane NE, Sanchez S, Modin GW et al. Parathyroid hormone treatment can reverse corticosteroid-induced osteoporosis. Results of a randomized controlled clinical trial. *J Clin Invest* 1998;102:1627–33.

Neer R, Hayes A, Rao A, Finkelstein J. Effects of parathyroid hormone, alendronate, or both on bone density in osteoporotic postmenopausal women. *J Bone Miner Res* 2002;17(suppl 1):S135.

Reid IR, Brown JP, Burckhardt P et al. Intravenous zoledronic acid in postmenopausal women with low bone mineral density. *N Engl J Med* 2002;346:653–61.

Rittmaster RS, Bolognese M, Ettinger MP et al. Enhancement of bone mass in osteoporotic women with parathyroid hormone followed by alendronate. *J Clin Endocrinol Metab* 2000;85:2129–34.

Useful addresses

UK

British Menopause Society
4–6 Eton Place
Marlow
Bucks SL7 2QA
Tel: +44 (0)1628 890199
www.thebms.org.uk

Menopause Matters
www.menopausematters.co.uk

National Osteoporosis Society
Manor Farm, Skinners Hill
Camerton, Bath BA2 0PJ
Tel: +44 (0)1761 471771
Helpline: 0845 450 0230
(Mon–Fri 9 AM–5 PM)
info@nos.org.uk
www.nos.org.uk

Women's Health
www.womenshealthlondon.org.uk

Women's Health Concern
4–6 Eton Place
Marlow
Bucks SL7 2QA
Tel: +44 (0)1628 478 473
Helpline: 0845 123 2319
(Mon, Wed and Thu 10–12 AM)
www.womens-health-concern.org

USA

National Osteoporosis Foundation
1232 22nd Street NW
Washington, DC 20037-1202
Tel: +1 202 223 2226/
+1 800 231 4222
www.nof.org

National Women's Health Resource Center
157 Broad Street
Suite 106 Red Bank
NJ 07701
Tel: +1 877 986 9472 (toll-free)
info@healthywomen.org
www.healthywomen.org

The North American Menopause Society
5900 Landerbrook Drive
Suite 390, Mayfield Heights
OH 44124
Tel: +1 440 442 7550
info@menopause.org
www.menopause.org

Women's Health Initiative
nm9o@nih.gov (WHI staff)
www.nhlbi.nih.gov/whi

International

Australasian Menopause Society
PO Box 676, Wynnum
Qld 1478
Tel: +61 (0)7 4642 1603
ams@netlink.com.au
www.menopause.org.au

European Menopause and Andropause Society
Kenes International
PO Box 1726
1–3, rue de Chantepoulet
CH-1211, Geneva 1
Switzerland
Tel: +41 22 908 04 82
info@emasononline.org
www.emasonline.org

European Mens' Health Forum
www.emhf.org

International Bone and Mineral Society
2025 M Street, NW, Suite 800
Washington, DC 20036-3309
Tel: +1 202 367 1121
info@ibmsonline.org
www.ibmsonline.org

International Menopause Society
PO Box 687, Wray, Lancaster,
LA2 8WY, UK
Tel: +44 (0)1524 221190
www.imsociety.org

International Osteoporosis Foundation
9, rue Juste-Olivier
CH-1260 Nyon
Switzerland
Tel: +41 22 994 0100
www.iofbonehealth.org
A full list of national osteoporosis societies is available at:
www.iofbonehealth.org/patients-public/osteoporosis-societies-worldwide.html

National Osteoporosis Foundation of South Africa
PO Box 481
Bellville Cape Town 7535
Tel: +27 (0)21 931 7894
www.osteoporosis.org.za

Osteoporosis Australia
Level 1, 52 Parramatta Road
Glebe 2037, NSW
Tel: +61 (02) 9518 8140
www.osteoporosis.org.au

Osteoporosis Canada
1090 Don Mills Road
Suite 301 Toronto
Ontario M3C 3R6
Tel: +1 416 696 2663
Toll-free: 1 800 463 6842
(Mon–Fri, 9 AM to 5 PM)
www.osteoporosis.ca

Index

acute phase reactions 69
adverse effects *see* side
    effects
age
    bone mass 7, 14, 20–1
    epidemiology 8–10, 49
alcohol abuse 44
alendronate 53, 54, 60–2,
    86, 87, 93
AMG 162 93
analgesia 29–30, 57
anticonvulsants 23
athletes 20
atrial fibrillation 69

back braces 30
back pain 25, 26
biochemical markers 41, 55,
    58, 90–1
bisphosphonates 53, 54,
    60–70
    combination therapy 93–4
    in men 62, 64, 87–8
    for steroid-induced
        osteoporosis 86, 87
bone cancer, metastatic 23,
    28, 60
bone marrow 21
bone mass
    acquisition and loss 7,
        12–23, 56, 91
    biochemical markers of
        change 41, 55, 58, 90–1
    BMD measurement
        techniques 32–9, 90
    effect of treatment 52, 54,
        56, 57, 58, 74
    low BMD as a risk factor
        12, 45–6
bone multicellular units
    (BMUs) 14
bone scans 27, 43
BONE trial 64–5
breast cancer 71, 73

calcaneus, imaging of 38–9,
    90

calcitonin 30, 53, 54, 74
calcitriol 53, 54
calcium
    deficiency 21
    hypercalcemia caused by
        PTH peptides 82, 93
    supplements 17, 69, 74–6,
        87, 88
cardiovascular disease 69,
    71, 73
clinical presentation 25–9,
    31, 32, 39
collagen crosslinks 41, 90
Colles' fractures 25, 29, 61
compliance 53, 58
computed tomography 38,
    90
cortical bone 14, 29
costs of healthcare provision
    7, 54, 92, 94
counseling 57–8

dental disease 70
diagnosis 43
    biochemical markers 41,
        90–1
    bone densitometry 32–9,
        90
    clinical examination 25–9,
        32, 39
    future trends 90–1
    secondary causes 32, 41–4
diet 23, 57
DIVA trial 66
dowager's hump 27
dual-energy X-ray
    absorptiometry (DXA) 27,
    34–8

economic issues 7, 54, 92, 94
efficacy of treatment 52–3
    alendronate 60–2, 86, 87–8
    calcitonin 74
    calcium +/– vitamin D 74–6
    etidronate 69, 86
    HRT 72
    ibandronate 64–6

efficacy of treatment
    continued
    raloxifene 70
    risedronate 62–4, 86, 88
    strontium ranelate 78–80
    teriparatide 81–2
    zoledronate 66–8
endometrial cancer 70, 72
epidemiology 7–10, 49, 87,
    90
esophagitis 62
estrogen 18–19
    HRT 53, 54, 72–3
ethnicity 9
etidronate 53, 69, 86
etiology 12, 17–23, 44,
    45–50, 85–6, 87
exercise 17, 57

falls 12, 29, 48, 57, 76
femoral fractures
    head/neck *see* hip
        fractures
    shaft 70
FIT trial 60–1
forearm fractures
    efficacy of treatment 61
    epidemiology 8, 9
    presentation 25, 29
fractures
    epidemiology 7–10
    management 29–30
    morbidity 7, 30–1
    presentation 25–9, 31,
        39–40
    risk factors 12, 17–23, 44,
        45–50, 85–6, 87
    see also efficacy of
        treatment
FRAX risk assessment
    algorithm 46–7, 49–50
future trends 90–4

gastrointestinal side effects
    62, 69
gender 7–10, 87
genetics 15–17, 91

glucocorticoid-induced
osteoporosis 21–2, 44, 62,
64, 85–7, 93
glucocorticoids, as analgesics
30

healthcare provision 94
heel, imaging of 38–9, 90
hip, BMD measurement 37
hip fractures
efficacy of treatment 53,
61, 63, 63–4, 79
epidemiology 8, 9, 45, 85
presentation 28–9, 30
hip protectors 57
HORIZON trial 66–7
hormone replacement
therapy (HRT) 53, 54,
72–3
humerus 29
hypercalcemia 82, 93
hyperparathyroidism 21, 82
hypogonadism 44, 87
see also menopause

ibandronate 53, 64–6
imaging
bone densitometry 34–9,
90
radiography 26–7, 39–40
immunosuppressants 23, 87

kyphoplasty 30
kyphosis 27, 32

lifestyle 23, 30, 57
lipoprotein receptor-related
protein 5 (LRP5) signaling
pathway 15–16
lipoxygenase pathway 16–17

magnetic resonance imaging
(MRI) 90
management 59, 75, 83, 88
anabolic agents 78–83, 86,
93
antiresorptive agents
60–76, 86, 87–8, 92, 93–4
choice of treatment 46,
52–4, 92
fractures 29–30

management continued
future trends 92–4
in men 62, 64, 87–8
monitoring 52, 55, 58
non-pharmacological 30,
56–8
steroid-induced
osteoporosis 86–7, 93
men
epidemiology 8–10, 44, 87
treatment 62, 64, 87–8
menopause 18–19, 71
MOBILE trial 66
MORE trial 70
myeloma 23, 43, 60

osteoblasts 14, 21
osteoclasts 14, 74
osteocytes 14
osteogenesis imperfecta 32
osteomalacia 43
osteonecrosis of the jaw
69–70
osteopenia 25, 28, 33, 39
osteoporosis
pseudoganglioma
syndrome 16
osteosarcoma 82

pain (in the back) 25, 26
pain relief 29–30, 57
parathyroid hormone (PTH)
calcium and 21, 74
PTH 1-84 53, 82, 93
PTHrp 93
teriparatide (PTH 1-34) 53,
54, 80–2, 86, 88, 93
pathophysiology 12–23, 85,
87
pelvis 29
physical activity 17, 57
physiotherapy 30, 57
pregnancy 87
progestogens 72
PTH see parathyroid
hormone

quantitative computed
tomography (QCT) 38, 90
quantitative ultrasound
(QUS) 38–9

radiography 26–7, 39–40
radius see forearm
raloxifene 53, 54, 70–2
RANK ligand inhibitors
93–4
ribs 29
risedronate 53, 62–4, 86, 88
risk assessment algorithm
(FRAX) 46–7, 49–50
risk factors 12, 17–23, 44,
45–50, 85–6, 87

screening 38–9, 49–50, 90,
92
sCT (salmon calcitonin) 30,
53, 54, 74
selective estrogen-receptor
modulators (SERMs) 53,
54, 70–2, 92
service provision 94
side effects 53–4
bisphosphonates 62, 66,
69, 69–70
calcitonin 74
HRT 73
raloxifene 70–1
strontium ranelate 80
teriparatide 82
SOTI trial 78
spinal BMD measurement
34–8
spinal fractures
epidemiology 8, 9, 85
management of fractures
29–30
presentation 25, 26–7,
39–40
see also efficacy of treatment
steroids see estrogen;
glucocorticoids
stroke 71, 73
strontium ranelate 53, 54,
78–80
support groups 57–8

T-scores 32–3, 38, 87
tamoxifen 92
tartrate-resistant acid
phosphatase 5b 91
teriparatide (PTH 1-34) 53,
54, 80–2, 86, 88, 93

thromboembolism 71, 73
thyroid disease 23
tibia 29
tolerability of treatment *see* side effects
trabecular bone 14, 29
treatment *see* management
TROPOS trial 79

UK, epidemiology 7, 8
ultrasound 38–9
USA, epidemiology 7, 8

vertebral fractures *see* spinal fractures
vertebroplasty 30
vitamin D 21, 74–6, 87, 88

Wnt signaling pathway 15–16
women
at the menopause 18–19, 71
epidemiology 7–10
premenopausal 87

women *continued*
treatment *see* management
Women's Health Initiative study 72
wrist fractures 25, 29, 61

X-rays
DXA 27, 34–8
radiography 26–7, 39–40

Z-scores 34
zoledronate 53, 66–9

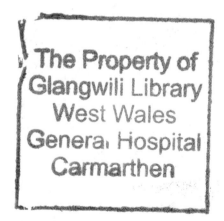